Angélica R. A. Leonídio
Maria Auxiliadora Andrade

Salmonella sp. in broiler production

Angélica R. A. Leonídio
Maria Auxiliadora Andrade

Salmonella sp. in broiler production

Main sources of infection for poultry and feed additives used to control them

ScienciaScripts

Imprint

Cover image: www.ingimage.com

This book is a translation from the original published under ISBN 978-3-330-76145-2.

Publisher:
Sciencia Scripts
is a trademark of
Dodo Books Indian Ocean Ltd. and OmniScriptum S.R.L publishing group

120 High Road, East Finchley, London, N2 9ED, United Kingdom
Str. Armeneasca 28/1, office 1, Chisinau MD-2012, Republic of Moldova, Europe
Managing Directors: Ieva Konstantinova, Victoria Ursu
info@omniscriptum.com

Printed at: see last page
ISBN: 978-620-8-37191-3

Index

CHAPTER 1

Introduction

Infectious diseases in animals, particularly zoonoses, are taking on greater prominence in public health and the global economic scenario. In this context, products from the poultry chain are important agents of food-borne infections, caused mainly by bacteria of the Salmonella genus, especially paratyphoid bacteria, which adapt easily to a large number of animal hosts, including humans.

Due to the increase in global food demand, it has been necessary to increase animal production. In the current farming model, birds or the end product can become infected with Salmonella from a variety of sources, such as replacement birds, the hatchery, the production environment, the slaughterhouse, wild and domestic animals, failures in biosecurity, management, facilities, food, among others. In large-scale intensive farming, microorganisms such as Salmonella can easily spread once they are introduced to farms. As they do not have specific hosts, it is almost impossible to eradicate the bacteria from the rearing environment or eliminate them from the products of contaminated animals (CARDOSO & TESSARI, 2008; FREITAS NETO et al. 2010).

The international commercialisation of food of animal origin is subject to sanitary barriers, since importing countries block the entry of products contaminated with pathogens, thus avoiding infection of consumers. Thus, the high health standards of Brazilian poultry farms are one of the main factors that affect the quality of the chicken meat produced, especially in the South, Southeast and Centre-West regions (MOREIRA et al., 2008).

In order to reduce the infection rate of animals and productivity losses associated with salmonellosis, alternative additives such as prebiotics, probiotics, symbiotics, organic acids and phytogenic compounds are constantly being studied to determine to what extent they can or cannot be used, and under what conditions they are viable.

In view of the above, this book aims to address the main sources of Salmonella infection for broilers in the production environment and in pre-slaughter operations, as well as listing the main feed additives that can be used to control salmonellosis in poultry.

CHAPTER 2

Salmonella sp.

The Salmonella genus belongs to the Enterobacteriaceae family and is made up of Gram-negative, non-spore-forming, aerobic or facultative anaerobic bacilli, most of which have flagella. They ferment glucose and other sugars and decarboxylate amino acids, chemical reactions that are important for characterising the genus and differentiating biotypes. They grow at temperatures between 5 and 45°C, but their comfort zone is between 37 and 40°C (ANDREATTI FILHO, 2007).

According to the CDC (2011), this genus is subdivided into two species, enterica and bongori. The Salmonella enterica species is subdivided into six species that are designated by taxonomic names, which can be abbreviated by Roman numerals, as shown in the table below:

TABLE 01 - Distribution of *Salmonella enterica* subspecies

Salmonella enterica - Subspecies	
1	*Salmonella enteric* subsp. enter/ca
II	*Salmomella enterica* subsp. sa/amae
IIIa	*Salmonella enteric* subsp. *azoonae*
IIIb	*Salmonella entaríco* subsp. *diarízonae*
IV	*Salmonelle enteuien* subsp. *Ouutnaee*
VI	*Salmonella enterica* subsp. *indica*

Source: Adapted from CDC (2011)

Serotyping is a method used to differentiate Salmonella isolates beyond subspecies levels (CDC, 2011). The classification system used is Kauffmann-White, which is based on the various antigenic structures found on the cell surface. These structures are the cell envelope or capsule ("Vi" capsular antigen), the cell wall ("O" somatic antigens) and the flagella ("H" flagellar antigens) (FERREIRA & CAMPOS, 2008).

The somatic antigen O is a carbohydrate, the outermost component of the cell surface containing lipopolysaccharide (LPS). It consists of a polymer made up of O subunits with four to six carbons. The variation between O antigens is due to the different types of sugars that make up their subunits and the nature of the bonds between the sugars and between the O subunits.

The H antigen is the filamentous portion of the bacterial flagellum, made up of protein subunits called flagellins. The antigenically variable portion of the flagellin is the central region, which is exposed on the surface of the flagellum. The Salmonella genus is the only one that can express two different flagellin antigens, referred to as Phase 1 and Phase 2 antigens. Their expression is coordinated so that only one flagellar antigen is expressed at a time (CDC, 2008).

The serovars of Salmonella enterica subspecies I cause disease in various warm-blooded animals and, even though they share genetic similarities, they vary in terms of host specificity. Some serovars are more limited, while others are capable of causing disease in several animals. For example, Salmonella Tiphy causes disease only in humans, while Salmonella Typhimurium causes gastroenteritis and rarely septicaemia in humans and lethal diarrhoea in cattle (ERREIRA & CAMPOS, 2008).

Infections caused by the Salmonella genus began to be reported in poultry in 1899 and have been intensively investigated ever since. In poultry, they cause a variety of acute and chronic diseases, being clinically classified into: pulorosis (caused by Salmonella Pullorum), fowl typhoid (caused by Salmonella Gallinarum) and paratyphoid infections. The third form of the disease is of greater importance in public and animal health, since it is frequently isolated in poultry products. Most of the paratyphoid serovars can colonise the gastrointestinal tract of birds without causing clinical disease, however, the Enteritidis and Typhimurium serovars can cause illness and food poisoning in humans (WRAY et al., 1998; CARDOSO & TESSARI, 2008).

CHAPTER 3

Salmonella sp. and public health

Poultry plays an important role as a vehicle of transmission in cases of human salmonellosis (WHO, 2002). The main foods involved in its transmission are eggs, poultry meat and their derivatives. Contamination of chicken carcasses can result from the presence of the bacteria in the rearing environment, which spreads during the slaughter operation if hygienic care is not taken (CARDOSO & TESSARI, 2008).

Many studies in Brazil have found the presence of Salmonella in chicken carcasses and their by-products. Analysing samples of chicken meat and by-products from the north-eastern region of the state of São Paulo, Carvalho & Cortez (2005) identified the presence of the microorganism in 13.3% (6/45) of carcasses, 25% (15/60) of mechanically separated meat (MSM), 16% (4/25) in sausages, 30% (6/20) of breasts and 13.3% (2/15) of thighs and drumsticks analysed. Moreira et al. (2008) also investigated the occurrence of Salmonella in chicken carcasses slaughtered in the state of Goiás and confirmed the presence of the bacteria in 14.32% (52/363) of them, where 11 serovars were isolated, with Salmonella Albany being the most frequently isolated.

Hall et al. (2009) collected 50 samples of raw chicken meat from nine commercial establishments in Botucatu-SP in order to determine the microbiological quality of this product. The analysis revealed that 8% of the samples were contaminated with Salmonella sp. (4/50). In the study by Borsoi et al. (2010), the authors found the frequency of Salmonella isolation in 12.2% (22/180) of chicken carcasses collected in Rio Grande do Sul, in which the Enteritidis serovar was the most present.

Salmonellosis control is a public health challenge due to the emergence/resurgence of serovars in different areas, both in developing and developed countries. Carrier animals are important epidemiological factors, due to the absence of symptoms and the technical difficulty in detecting them before or during animal health inspection (TESSARI et al., 2012). Carrier birds become infected at a young age, when their immune system is not yet capable of eliminating the bacteria from the gastrointestinal tract, making systemic infection possible. When they don't die, they recover and can become carriers, transmitting the pathogen both horizontally and vertically during stressful periods (BERCHIERI JÚNIOR & FREITAS NETO, 2009).

When estimating the global number of gastroenteritis caused by Salmonella of the paratyphoid type, Majowicz et al. (2010) estimated that approximately 93.8 million cases of gastroenteritis occur annually worldwide, of which 155,000 patients die. The authors also found that 80.3 million cases were related to the consumption of contaminated food.

Recent data from a salmonellosis outbreak in the USA, where 195 people were infected with Salmonella serovars Infantis, Newport and Lille in 27 states. The infected people reported contact with live poultry from an Ohio hatchery (CDC, 2012).

Epidemiological data on FBD (Foodborne Diseases) in Brazil is limited (KOTTWITZ et al., 2010). The Ministry of Health recorded 8,663 outbreaks of FBD between 2000 and 2011. Of the reported cases, Salmonella sp. was responsible for 1,660 outbreaks, and in 4,148 the responsible microorganism was not identified. Therefore, the number of cases associated with this pathogen could be much higher (BRASIL, 2012).

In a study carried out by Nadvorny et al. (2004), outbreaks caused by Salmonella sp. in the year 2000 in the state of Rio Grande do Sul and the main related foods were analysed. The authors found that foods prepared with eggs were involved in 72.2 per cent of the outbreaks and chicken meat in 11.4 per cent, showing that 83.6 per cent of the cases involved products from the poultry chain.

An outbreak of 94 cases of Salmonella infections in 2008 in the metropolitan area of Adelaide, Australia, was analysed by Fearnley et al. (2011). The researchers found that in the days leading up to the outbreak, 62.8 per cent of patients reported eating chicken meat. Of the 31 serovars isolated in the outbreak, Salmonella Typhimurium was identified in 61.7 per cent.

According to Freitas Neto et al. (2010), despite the strong link between the consumption of food of animal origin and human salmonellosis, people can become infected through other routes, such as cross-contamination in domestic and commercial kitchens, through contact with other people and animals (especially dogs, cats and reptiles), as well as the ingestion of vegetables and fruit. Recently, an outbreak caused by Salmonella Braenderup, reported in 15 US states, where 127 people were infected and 33 hospitalised, was linked to the consumption of mangoes from Mexico (CDC, 2012).

According to Cardoso & Carvalho (2006), outbreaks caused by Salmonella sp. are likely to occur much more frequently than they are reported or diagnosed, since various foods can carry the microorganism, and both handlers and consumers are unaware of the possible risks involved in their preparation.

CHAPTER 4

Sources of Salmonella sp. infection in the production environment

4.1 Hatchery

The contamination and penetration of Salmonella sp. in hatching eggs can determine an important link in the transmission of this pathogen to growing birds, processed carcasses and, eventually, to the consumer (PRADHAN et al., 2005). According to Cox et al. (2000), the presence of this bacterium in hatching eggs has been identified as a critical point in the contamination of broilers with this bacterium.

According to Cox et al. (2000), there are two main lines of thought regarding the introduction of Salmonella sp. into hatching eggs. In the vertical transmission theory, the bacterium originates from an infected hen. The theory of horizontal transmission states that the pathogen invades the egg through the shell, shortly after laying. In fact, both mechanisms are possibly involved.

In poultry, Salmonella Enteritidis is able to colonise the hen's egg-laying canal, causing contamination of the membrane surrounding the yolk during egg formation. However, eggs can also be contaminated by contact with the environment, during or after laying, during their transit through the cloaca. The microorganism is deposited and then penetrates through the shell structures. In this way, the capacity for vertical and horizontal transmission of Salmonella has spread widely in the poultry industry (CARDOSO & TESSARI, 2008).

The egg has several physical barriers that make it difficult for microorganisms to invade. Even if they manage to successfully penetrate the shell, their survival and multiplication inside the egg can be jeopardised. The viscosity of the albumen ensures that the microorganism remains localised, and together with the chalaza and albuminous sac, prevents it from coming into contact with the yolk. In addition, the presence of lysozymes in albumin hydrolyse the peptide glycans present in the bacterial cell wall (SESTI & ITO, 2009).

Pradhan et al. (2005), using eggs contaminated with Salmonella Typhimurium, observed that the microbial load decreased during the first 10 days of incubation due to the migration of bacteria from the eggshell to the allantoic fluid, which has antimicrobial activity. The authors also found that after 17 days of incubation, the microbial population in the shell, shell membrane and yolk was lower compared to the first 10 days of incubation, as a result of migration and colonisation of the chick embryos' gastrointestinal tract.

In the study by Andrade et al. (2009), the invasive capacity of Salmonella Enteritidis was assessed in embryonated eggs from two broiler strains. The eggs were inoculated on the shell using contaminated hands and in the albumen to simulate horizontal and vertical transmission, respectively. The birds' meconium was collected and it was found that 10% (3/30) of the birds from the ISA Label strain and 50% (15/30) from the Ross strain that were inoculated on the shell had the bacteria in their excreta. For eggs inoculated via albumen, the isolation frequencies were 26.7 per cent (8/30) for the ISA Label strain and 76.8 per cent (23/30) for the Ross strain. The authors concluded that both the strain and the route of inoculation influenced the number of chicks infected with the bacteria.

The presence of Salmonella sp. in the nests, transport lorry or incubation environment can lead to egg contamination (COX et al., 2000). Kim et al. (2007) detected the presence of Salmonella Enteritidis in the nests and dust on the walls of a broiler breeder farm. In the study conducted by Osman et al. (2010), it was observed that the highest frequencies of Salmonella isolation (18.4%) were in the boxes transporting the chicks. The most isolated serovar was Newport, followed by Enteritidis, Shubra and Agona. Moraes (2010) also assessed the presence of the bacteria in transport box linings and found it in 9.4% of the 32 samples collected. Marin et al. (2011) detected Salmonella in 32 per cent of chick transport boxes on farms in eastern Spain.

According to Andreatti Filho (2007), when eggs that are contaminated, either on the shell or inside, reach the hatchery, the transmission of the bacteria is favoured. Egg fragments, such as the shell and yolk, the chicks themselves, their feathers and meconium, are highly contaminating sources. From contaminated incubators, Salmonella can spread through the air, contaminating various sectors of the hatchery.

Several studies in Brazil have reported the presence of Salmonella in day-old chicks. Gambiragi et al. (2003), using the rapid serum agglutination method on 300 venous blood samples from day-old chicks from the metropolitan region of Fortaleza - Ceará, found that 100 samples were positive for Salmonella. Rocha et al. (2003) observed that 3% (6/198) of the samples from the organ pool of chicks from three integrating companies in the state of Goiás were infected with the bacteria. Perdoncini et al. (2011) also isolated the bacteria from the liver of 2.32% (3/129) of chicks marketed for non-industrial production in Santa Catarina.

4.2 Ration

Feed contaminated with Salmonella has been the most common source of introduction of new strains of the bacterium into the animal production chain and from where it is subsequently distributed to other sectors through the movement of animals (OIE, 2010). The increase in cases of food-borne salmonellosis in Western Europe between the 1980s and 1990s led to the creation of new control measures, firstly in the poultry industry and later in pig and beef production.

Contamination of feed with microbiological and chemical agents can affect the health, performance and welfare of animals, as well as influencing the safety of food of animal origin and negatively affecting human health. Therefore, safe feed is an essential prerequisite for the efficient production of safe food (FLACHOWSKY, 2012).

Feed can contain a diverse microbiota that is acquired from multiple environmental sources, such as dust, soil, water, plants and insects. Raw materials can be contaminated at any time during cultivation, harvesting, processing, storage and delivery. The microbiological diversity found in food depends on water activity, oxygen tension, pH, nutrient composition and moisture content. Some microorganisms can adapt to the scarcity of free water and can actively grow on grains. However, the majority must have strategies to survive in the feed until there are favourable conditions for their development (MACIOROWSKI et al., 2007).

Feed and its raw materials, especially those of animal origin, often show high contamination rates by

Salmonella sp. (SILVA & DUARTE, 2002). According to Radcliff (2006), contamination of raw materials is the result of poor hygiene during processing and contact with the faeces of rodents, insects and birds.

Morita et al. (2005) in their study on possible sources of Salmonella contamination in a feed mill, detected the bacteria in all the vectors investigated: operators, machine surfaces, factory floors, dust and rodents. In particular, high concentrations of the microorganism were isolated from the floor of the processing area, due to its high oil content. Rodents in the same area were also highly contaminated, with 46.4 per cent isolation. The percentage of Salmonella detected on the operators' shoes was the highest of all the vectors, revealing the importance of restricting the movement of people between the clean and dirty areas of the factory, preventing the spread of the pathogen.

Some strains occasionally isolated from feed mills can survive in the industry for several years. One hypothesis for this persistence is the formation of biofilms on the machines, which protect the bacteria from stresses such as disinfection (VESTBY et al., 2009). In the study by Torres et al. (2011), 3,844 feed samples were collected from 523 Spanish factories to check for the presence of Salmonella. The presence of the bacteria was detected in 185 samples, 3.5 per cent of which were feed, 3.3 per cent ingredients and 12.5 per cent mill dust.

For this reason, raw materials of animal origin have been removed from broiler feed formulations as a method of controlling the agent (SILVA & DUARTE, 2002). Ingredients such as feather and viscera meal are responsible for a process known as "*Salmonella* recycling" (SILVA, 2005). In the study by Moraes (2010), the presence of Salmonella sp. was verified in samples of offal, meat, blood and feather meal. The author detected the presence of the bacteria in 10.5% of the samples analysed. The frequency in meat meal was 12%, in blood meal 6.8%, in feathers 4.3% and in viscera 14.6%.

4.3 Aviary litter

Poultry litter is a covering that is 5 to 10 cm thick and is placed on the floor of the poultry house. It can be made up of various types of material, such as pine sawdust or wood shavings, eucalyptus, hardwood, rice husks, sugarcane bagasse, corn cobs or straw. This device has the function of providing comfort for the birds, enabling the quality of the carcasses to be preserved, reducing the incidence of injuries in the breast, knee and plantar cushion regions, and can be reused in up to eight production batches (OLIVEIRA & CARVALHO, 2002; LUCCA et al., 2012).

Poultry is an important source of contamination for the dissemination of enterobacteria into the environment. Their litter can contain a diverse population of microorganisms, some of which are potentially pathogenic to birds, humans or both (CARVALHO et al. 2001).

Reusing poultry litter is a common practice in the Brazilian poultry industry due to two important aspects: reducing production costs and environmental sustainability (ROLL et al., 2011). Reused litter can be a residual source of Salmonella and can transfer the bacteria to the next production cycles. Procedures for reusing litter vary between countries, but there is worldwide concern about the possible transmission of pathogens between flocks (CHINIVASAGAM et al., 2012).

The microbiology of litter is very diverse due to the constant deposition of faecal matter, secretions and scaling from the birds, as well as fungi and bacteria present in the environment (VIEIRA, 2011). Microbial growth in litter is inherent to poultry production and can be minimised, but not eliminated (FIORENTIN, 2005).

Many studies in Brazil have found a low presence of Salmonella sp. in trawl feeds collected in poultry sheds. In the study by Andreatti Filho et al. (2009), 806 trawl suabes were collected and in 22 of them (2.7%) the bacterium was isolated. Boni et al. (2011) found the presence of Salmonella in only 3.73% of the 134 trawl samples collected. Roll et al. (2011) also found the presence of the bacteria in only 2.5%, 5.27% and 2.08% in 2008, 2009 and 2010, respectively.

4.4 Mechanical loaders

There are many important biological carriers in the transmission of Salmonella sp. to poultry. Domestic and wild animals, including birds, rodents, insects and man himself can spread/maintain the bacteria over long periods in the rearing environment (ANDREATTI FILHO, 2007).

Farms have large quantities of high-quality food, manure and dead birds. The shed, which is enclosed, heated and protected from the sun and rain, provides a place for these animals to live and multiply (OVIEDO-RONDÓN, 2008).

Rats and mice are recognised as sources of Salmonella and are attracted to poultry farms by the abundance of easily accessible food. Rats have been shown to be important vectors of Salmonella Enteritidis in the current epidemic (WRAY et al., 1998). Through their secretions and faeces, the bacteria come into contact with raw materials and poultry feed (ANDREATTI FILHO, 2007).

In recent years, the involvement of wild birds has become evident, as they can become infected and also spread the bacteria mechanically through their feet (WRAY et al., 1998). Salmonella Typhimurium is commonly found in the intestines of these birds, which become infected by eating sick prey or by faecal contamination (TIZARD, 2004).

In the study by Hughes et a. (2008), they typed Salmonella isolates from wild birds in the north of England between 2005 and 2006. The authors confirmed Salmonella Typhimurium in 29 of the 32 samples. Mirzae et al. (2010) isolated the bacterium from 3.8 per cent (18/470) of the viscera samples of sparrows caught in the Tehran region, the capital of Iran. Among the isolates, the serovars Typhimurium and Enteritidis were the most frequent.

In layer manure and chicken litter, house flies (Musca domestica) and sand flies (califoridae and sarcofagidae) multiply easily (PEDROSO-DE-PAIVA, 2000). In their study, Holt et al. (2007) placed house fly fleas in the houses of laying hens inoculated with Salmonella Enteritidis and then analysed the contamination of the insect by the bacteria. The authors observed that after 48 hours, 45 to 50 per cent of the flies had detectable amounts of the pathogen in their bodies.

Mealybugs (Alphitobius diaperinus) feed on faeces, carcasses, fungi, grain and stored flour. These insects are carriers and vectors of pathogens due to their feeding habits. By feeding on dead and dying birds, they increase their chances of assuming the role of mechanical vectors of pathogens. Feeding on weak birds also increases their weakness (PEDROSO-DE-PAIVA, 2000).

When investigating the frequency of isolation of Salmonella sp. in snail samples, Moraes (2010) found that 12.5 per cent of the insects were positive for the bacterium. Unlike the results found by Chernaki-Leffer et al. (2002), who did not isolate Salmonella from the insects. In the study by Segabinazi et al. (2005), the authors isolated the bacterium in only 0.37% of the rattlesnake samples.

Farm workers can mechanically carry Salmonella from one unit to another through contaminated clothing, footwear and hands, and can also be carriers of the disease and excrete the bacteria while working, infecting the birds (WRAY et al., 1998). In the study by Marin et al. (2011), the authors isolated Salmonella in 19.7% of 61 boot swabs from farm workers in Spain.

CHAPTER 5

Main feed additives used to control Salmonella sp. in broilers

SARC (Secretary of Rural Support and Cooperativism) Order° 013 of 30/11/2004 aims to establish the basic procedures that must be adopted for assessing the safety of use, registration and marketing of additives used in products intended for animal feed. This decree defines an additive as: "a substance, micro-organism or formulated product, intentionally added to products, which is not normally used as an ingredient, whether or not it has nutritional value and which improves the characteristics of products intended for animal feed or animal products, improves the performance of healthy animals and fulfils nutritional needs"... (BRASIL, 2009).

According to the same ordinance, to be considered an additive, the product must be indispensable as a component of feed, have a positive influence on the characteristics of animal products, "be used in the quantity strictly necessary to obtain the desired effect" and be authorised and registered with the Ministry of Agriculture, Livestock and Supply (MAPA).

Among the various types of additives, zootechnical additives are designed to have a positive influence on improving animal performance. This category of additives includes the following functional groups: digestive (enzymes), intestinal flora balancers (probiotics, prebiotics and acidifiers), performance modulators (antibiotics).

4.5 Antibiotic growth modulators (AMDs)

Antibiotics have always been widely used for decades in animal production (HUYGHEBAERT et al., 2011). The history of the use of antibiotics in animal feed began with the isolation of vitamin B12. In the 1940s, poultry production boomed in the United States. However, animal protein sources for feed had become scarce and the large supply of plant-based proteins meant that they had to be replaced. Animal proteins contained an unknown factor that was necessary for the growth of chickens and pigs. Researchers then isolated vitamin B12 and assumed that this was the factor.

They later realised that the promoting effect was not the vitamin, but the antibiotic produced by certain fungi present in the feed (JONES & RICKET, 2003; DIBNER & RICHARDS, 2005).

Between 1960 and 2000, world pig production doubled and poultry production almost quadrupled. During this period, much of the feed offered to these production animals contained AMD (MILLET, 2011). These agents are also called zootechnical or production additives. Their effects on productivity translate into: increased weight gain; a reduction in the time needed to reach the ideal weight for slaughter; increased feed efficiency, a reduction in the amount of feed consumed by the animal, as well as the prevention of infectious pathologies and a reduction in mortality (PALERMO NETO, 2006).

The mechanisms of action of AMDs are focussed on the intestine. Four main mechanisms are proposed to explain their beneficial action: 1) they inhibit subclinical infections, reducing the metabolic costs of the immune system; 2) they reduce the production of metabolic depressants, such as ammonia produced by microorganisms; 3) they reduce the microbial use of nutrients and, 4) they increase the absorption of nutrients by the animal, since the intestinal wall is thinner due to the incorporation of AMD in the feed (NIEWOLD, 2007).

AMDs are used in dosages much lower than the Minimum Inhibitory Concentration (MIC) that is recommended for controlling pathogens (NIEWOLD, 2007). Their continuous use at low concentrations can induce antibiotic resistance in most bacteria (AARESTRUP, 2001; TEUBER, 2001). Due to the emergence of microorganisms that are resistant to antibiotics used to treat human and animal infections, the greatest concern is that cross-resistance may be induced between the bacteria that infect animals and those that are pathogenic to humans, even though this assumption has not been satisfactorily proven in scientific studies (ARAÚJO et al., 2007; HUYGHEBAERT et al., 2011).

Based on this questioning, the European Commission decided to phase out and finally ban the use of AMD in animal feed in January 2006. The ban on these drugs had a marked impact on animal production (HUYGHEBAERT et al., 2011; MILLET,

2011).

When discontinuing the use of antibiotics for non-therapeutic purposes, alternative options should be evaluated, which could be: a) stabilising the normal intestinal microbiota (e.g. pre- and probiotics); b) reducing the bacterial load in the digestive tract (e.g. organic acids); c) improving the vitality of enterocytes and villi (e.g. organic acids in vitamins); d) reducing the intake of immunosuppressive substances such as mycotoxins. organic acids); c) improving the vitality of enterocytes and villi (e.g. organic acids in vitamins); d) reducing the intake of immunosuppressive substances such as mycotoxins (e.g. sequestrants, alumino-silicates); e) optimising digestion (e.g. enzymes, herbal extracts); f) effectively controlling coccidiosis. Alternatives should also take into account that substitute products need to be safe, effective, low-cost and easy to use, without forgetting that there is a need to improve general production management in terms of air conditioning, hygiene of facilities, adequate nutrient supply in diets, purchase of genetic material from certified hatcheries with minimum avian health programmes (BELLAVER & SCHUERMMAN, 2004).

However, Huyghebaert et al. (2011) stated that no alternative product is likely to fully compensate for the withdrawal of AMDs from animal production. The authors also emphasise that some strategies will only help to partially compensate for, but not replace, antibiotics, acting through indirect mechanisms.

4.6Prebiotics

A prebiotic is defined as a non-digestible food ingredient that benefits the host by selectively affecting the intestinal microbiota and, consequently, favours the health of the host (GIBSON & ROBERFROID, 1995). According to Pessôa et al. (2012), prebiotics are ingredients that are not affected by digestive enzymes in the proximal portion of the GIT of monogastric animals, but which selectively stimulate the growth or activity of beneficial bacteria in the intestine.

Interest in utilising the intestinal microbial ecosystem has grown recently, and it has been used as a tool to improve animal and human health. In humans, the addition of prebiotics to the diet shows positive results in balancing the intestinal microbiota. A fully mature microbiota occupies all environmental niches and utilises almost all available nutrients, preventing pathogenic bacteria from occupying a position in the GIT. Advantages of using natural intestinal microbiota against pathogens include ease of application and low economic and labour costs. In addition, the use of one's own microbial ecosystem is seen as a "green" strategy in animal production (CALLAWAY et al., 2008; GAGGIA et al., 2010).

The main sources of prebiotics are some sugars, absorbable or not, fibres, peptides, proteins, sugar alcohols and oligosaccharides. Due to their chemical structure, these compounds are not absorbed in the upper part of the GIT or hydrolysed by digestive enzymes, so they manage to reach the colon and serve as a substrate for the microbiota. Non-digestible carbohydrates can be used as a substrate by bacteria, but not all are classified as prebiotics, as they can benefit the growth of both beneficial and pathogenic microorganisms (GIBSON & ROBERFROID, 1995; DIONÍSIO et al., 2002).

Gibson & Roberfroid (1995) defined some desirable characteristics of a prebiotic: it must not be metabolised or digested during its transit through the GIT; it must be taken up by beneficial intestinal bacteria, which will be stimulated to grow and/or become metabolically active; it must have the capacity to modify the intestinal microbiota in such a way as to favour the host and induce beneficial luminal or systemic effects on the host.

As prebiotics are not digested in the upper part of the intestine, they are fermented in the colon. When they are fermented, they promote an increase in volume as a result of stimulating microbial growth, as well as increasing the number of bowel movements. They are therefore classified as dietary fibres (ROBERFROID, 2002).

The most widely studied prebiotics in poultry nutrition are oligosaccharides, mainly mannan oligosaccharides (MOS), fructooligosaccharides (FOS) and glucoligosaccharides (GOS) (SILVA, 2010).

Some of the functions of prebiotics are shown in Table 02.

TABLE 02 - Intestinal functions attributed to prebiotics

Dietary fibres and gastrointestinal functions

Effects on the upper GIT	Resistance to digestion Delayed gastric emptying Increased oro-cecal transit time Reduced glucose absorption and low glycaemic index Hyperplasia of the small intestinal epithelium Stimulation of the secretion of hormonal intestinal peptides
Effects on the lower GIT	Acting as food for the colonic microbiota Acting as a substrate for fermentation Final fermentation products (mainly AGCC) Stimulation of saccharolytic fermentation Acidification of colon contents Hyperplasia of the colonic epithelium Stimulation of the secretion of hormonal peptides from the colon Effect on faeces production volume Regularisation of stool production (frequency and consistency) Accelerated caeco-anal transit

Source: Adapted from GAGGiA et al. (2010).

Oligosaccharides are generally extracted from the cell wall of vegetables such as chicory, onions, garlic, artichokes and asparagus, among others. They can also be extracted through the action of microbial enzymes in fermentation processes, using sucrose and starch as substrates. These compounds cannot be hydrolysed by digestive enzymes (FLEMMING, 2005).

MOS are derived from the cell wall of Saccharomyces cerevisiae yeasts and were introduced as feed additives for broiler chickens in 1993 (HOOGE et al., 2004; ALBINO et al., 2006). They have a high binding affinity with Gram-negative pathogenic bacteria that have oligosaccharide-specific type 1 fimbriae. Prebiotics are able to utilise the similarity between the binding sites of mannose-rich enterocytes and the mannan oligosaccharides added to the diet, reducing the attachment of these pathogens to the mucosa and facilitating their expulsion along with the excreta (FLEMMING, 2005).

Studies using MOS show that these compounds have the potential to stimulate the growth of beneficial bacteria as well as inhibiting pathogens such as Salmonella sp. and E. coli, improving the intestinal health and performance of poultry (SPRING et al., 2000; ALBINO et al., 2006; BAURHOO et al., 2007, CORRIGAN et al., 2011).

In their study, Kim et al. (2011) added prebiotics at different dosages to broiler feed and found that the populations of Clostridium perfringens and E. coli were reduced, while that of Lactobacillus showed significant growth.

Inulin and oligofructose are carbohydrates that are considered functional foods as they play a role in physiological and biochemical processes in the body. Inulin, oligofructose and FOS are chemically similar entities with the same nutritional properties (SAAD, 2006). These compounds have the property of stimulating the host's immune system and reducing levels of harmful bacteria (SILVA, 2010).

Bifidobacteria have fermentation specificity for FOS due to the production of the enzyme p-fructosidase (inulinases) (SAAD, 2006). By fermenting, these bacteria acidify the intestinal pH and thus inhibit the growth of pathogenic microorganisms (GIBSON & ROBERFROID, 1995). When investigating the growth of Salmonella Typhimurium in an in vitro caecal fermentation system, Donalson et al. (2007) observed that the bacteria were inhibited in the treatments in which FOS were added.

Lactulose is a disaccharide which, after ingestion, reaches the colon without undergoing many changes and is fermented by bifidobacteria, lactobacilli and other beneficial bacteria. The fatty acids produced during fermentation induce beneficial systemic and luminal effects (SILVA & NORNBERG, 2003). The study by Santana et al. (2012) assessed the influence of lactulose on animal performance and its ability to prevent colonisation by Salmonella Typhimurium in broilers inoculated orally. The researchers observed that the addition of lactulose improved the performance of the animals up to a week after inoculation, influenced the height of the intestinal villi and reduced the excretion of the pathogen in the faeces.

Prebiotics improved intestinal integrity in the study conducted by Silva et al. (2008), similar to the effect of AMD. However, Ramos et al. (2011) reported that the use of prebiotics decreased the height of the villi in the duodenum of the birds.

The intestinal environment is the site of interaction between microorganisms, food antigens and the immune system. Gut-associated lymphoid tissue (GALT) plays an important role in supplying immune system cells for defence against pathogens (BRISBIN et al., 2008). Studies suggest that Peyer's patches are sensitive to prebiotics, and the mechanisms of stimulation include: changes in the composition of the intestinal microbiota, immunological processes at the level of GALT, increased production of immunoglobulins and bacterial metabolites (SEIFERT & WATZL, 2007).

The use of prebiotics in animal feed, as a possible alternative to the use of AMDs, has shown contradictory results, while their use as an intestinal microbial modulator is effective. These compounds contribute to the establishment of bacteria such as bifidobacteria and lactobacilli, which may have beneficial effects on the host, to the detriment of harmful species (GAGGIA et al., 2010).

4.7 Probiotics

The term probiotic is derived from the Greek *probios* meaning "in favour of life". A probiotic is a living microorganism that has beneficial effects on the host's health, in addition to its inherent basic nutrition. The benefits associated with consuming whey and yoghurt have been known for centuries, but only in recent decades have probiotics been objectively evaluated as a method for preventing and treating diseases (MYERS, 2007).

Most of the concepts about the mechanism of action of probiotics are based on research carried out on mammals, many of which are not applicable to poultry. In these animals, it is estimated that the influence of the GIT microbiota on productivity and health is more evident than in other monogastric species (CORCIONIVOSCHI et al., 2010). Currently, probiotics are seen as production enhancers. By affecting the digestive microbiota in a positive way, they protect the organism against colonisation by harmful bacteria (GAGGIA et al., 2010).

The intestinal microbiota of birds is made up of numerous species of bacteria, forming a dynamic complex. Those that initially colonise the GIT tend to persist throughout the bird's life, becoming part of the resident microbial population. This population is formed shortly after hatching and increases during the first few weeks of life, and can be influenced by various factors, including age, diet and the use of antibiotics/probiotics (FURLAN et al., 2004; BRISBIN et al., 2008).

The natural microbiota of chicks is not always able to protect the organism from the invasion of pathogenic microorganisms. There is therefore a need for a defence strategy that can establish a symbiotic relationship between the host and beneficial microorganisms (FLEMMING, 2005).

Some desirable effects are expected from a probiotic, such as: the production of short and medium chain fatty acids, bacteriocins, reduction of intestinal pH, competition with enteropathogens for intestinal binding sites and stimulation of the immune response (HUME et al., 2011). Gaggia et al. (2010) also defined some expected characteristics and safety criteria for probiotics: non-toxic and non-pathogenic; precise taxonomic identification; natural inhabitant of the target species; production of microbial substances; antagonism to pathogenic bacteria; modulation of immune response; ability to exert at least one scientifically proven health-promoting property; genetic stability; receptivity of the strain and stability of the desired characteristics during processing, storage and supply; viability in high populations; desirable organoleptic and technological properties when included in industrial processes and colonisation, survival and being metabolically active at the site of action (resistance to gastric juice and bile; persistence in the GIT; adhesion to the epithelium or mucus and competition with the resident microbiota).

Some of the mechanisms of action of probiotics are outlined in Figure 01.

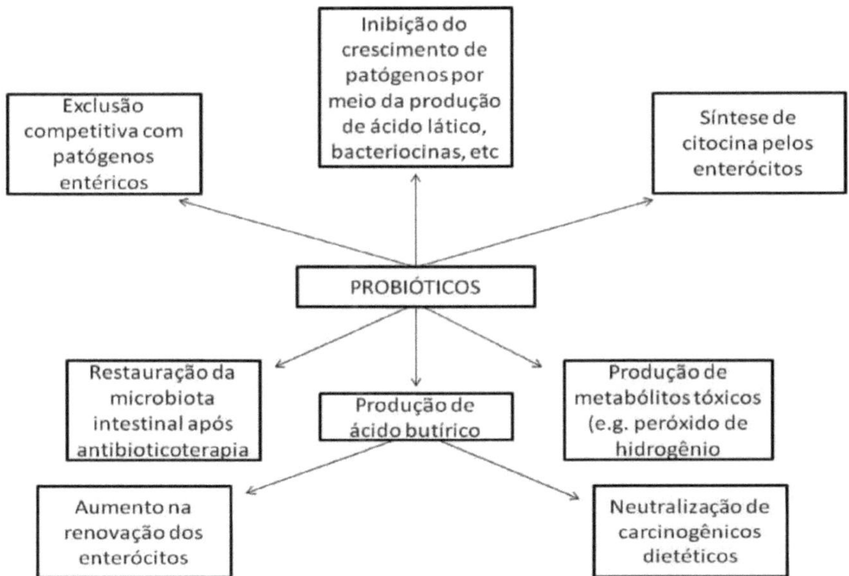

FIGURE 01 - Supposed mechanisms of action of probiotics

Source: Adapted from KAUR et al. (2002).

The term "competitive exclusion" is used to describe the inability of a microbial population to establish itself in the intestine due to the presence of another population. Competitive exclusion is an important tool in the prevention of intestinal diseases, especially those caused by E. coli and Salmonella sp. (CORCIONIVOSCHI et al., 2010).

In his review, Petri (2000) cited five main mechanisms of action of these products: 1) physical effect (barrier): the bacteria attach themselves to the intestinal mucosa, forming a protective barrier that prevents the colonisation of harmful bacteria; 2) biological effect: the anaerobic bacteria in the probiotic promote an environment of low oxygen tension, inhibiting the growth of enteropathogens; 3) chemical effect: the production of organic acids by bacteria causes a reduction in intestinal pH, discouraging colonisation by disease-causing microorganisms; 4) biochemical effect: production of bacteriocins; 5) nutritional effect: the bacteria in the probiotic cause a reduction in intestinal pH, discouraging colonisation by disease-causing microorganisms.

probiotics compete with enteropathogens for nutrients, reducing their colonisation in the gut.

When assessing the colonisation capacity of lactic acid bacteria and bifidobacteria and their activity in controlling three strains of Campylobacter jejuni in broilers, Santini et al. (2010) observed that the concentration of C. jejuni was reduced in the animals given Bifidobacterium longum, and its presence in the birds' excreta was high even after six days without being given. Carrying out in vitro tests with bacterial isolates from the GIT of chickens, Thirabunyanon & Thongwittaya (2012) found that Bacillus subtilis did not show cytotoxicity in intestinal cells and reduced the attachment of Salmonella Enteritidis to the intestinal surface.

As well as influencing intestinal functions such as motility and peristalsis, the intestinal microbiota also has important metabolic effects such as the production of short-chain fatty acids (SCFA) from fermentable carbohydrates, which become a source of energy for the colonic mucosa, promoting the growth and differentiation of enterocytes. The intestinal microbiota is also responsible for producing nutrients and vitamins, such as folic acid and vitamin K (SHANAHAN, 2002; QUIGLEY, 2010). Sen et al. (2012), when investigating the effect of dietary supplementation of Bacillus subtilis in broilers, found that there were improvements in bird performance and nutrient retention, as well as increasing the height of the villi in the duodenum and ileum and reducing the number of clostridia in the caecum. When evaluating the effect of different types of probiotics, Santos et al. (2013) observed that the height of the villi in the duodenum showed higher values when they received undefined microbiota.

One of the animal organism's main protective barriers to invasion by pathogenic microorganisms is gastric pH. In newly hatched chicks, the concentration of volatile fatty acids and the pH are not sufficient to suppress enteropathogens, and supplementing the diet with probiotics is a beneficial measure (FLEMMING, 2005). Bifidobacterium, Lactobacillus and Lactococcus, commonly known as lactic acid bacteria, are the microorganisms most commonly used as probiotics (BRISBIN et al., 2008).

The relationships established between the host and its microbiota can be commensal or symbiotic. The bacteria of the microbiota, as previously mentioned, are important in absorbing nutrients and preventing intestinal colonisation by harmful microorganisms. Therefore, recognition of the microbiota by the host's immune system is of fundamental importance (AURELI et al., 2011). Without this recognition, there would be an exacerbated immune response, posing a risk of excessive inflammation and intestinal damage (BRISBIN et al., 2008).

Faria Filho et al. (2006) evaluated the effectiveness of using probiotics as growth modulators in broiler feed, using a systematic review of studies published in Brazil between 1995 and 2005. The study showed that probiotics promoted better weight gain and feed conversion rates both in the initial phase (1 to 28 days) and throughout the rearing phase (1 to 35-48 days). The authors conclude that probiotics are a viable alternative to antibiotic growth modulators and that more studies are needed to identify any differences between probiotics commercially available in Brazil.

4.8 Symbiotics

Symbiotics are defined as a mixture of probiotics and prebiotics that act to benefit the host by improving the survival of microbial dietary supplements in the GIT. These compounds act by selectively stimulating the growth and/or metabolism of a certain group of microorganisms (GIBSON & ROBERFROID, 1995). This combination can improve the viability of probiotic microorganisms, since they use prebiotics as a substrate for fermentation, as well as improving the survival rate of probiotics during their passage through the GI tract, contributing to the stabilisation and/or enhancement of probiotic effects (AWAD et al., 2008; FALAKI et al., 2010).

The use of probiotics together with prebiotics is considered beneficial for the consumer organism, due to the fact that non-pathogenic bacteria establish themselves in the GIT by selectively stimulating their growth and by activating the metabolism of these bacteria that are beneficial to health, all as a result of a better intestinal environment provided by the prebiotics in the food (LIMA, 2006).

The benefits of using symbiotics include: 1) boosting the immune response; 2) increasing intestinal permeability; 3) balancing the intestinal microbiota; 4) improving the immune function of the intestinal barrier, and 5) regulating proinflammatory cytokines. The beneficial effects of symbiotics in controlling post-surgical complications in patients with liver disease have also been observed (USAMI et al., 2011).

Testing the inclusion of symbiotics in the feed of broiler chickens reared in conventional and alternative systems, Sartori et al. (2007) concluded that the use of symbiotics improved the performance of the birds at 42 days of age in both types of rearing system, but the addition of this additive to the feed increased production costs. Caramori Júnior et al. (2008) also found that symbiotic supplementation improved the birds' feed conversion. Falaki et al. (2010) reported that the addition of symbiotics to broiler diets improves their productive performance. When testing the effects of using probiotics, prebiotics and symbiotics on the intestinal morphometry of broilers challenged with Salmonella Enteritidis, Murate et al. (2013) observed that the symbiotic treatment showed a significant increase in jejunal villi.

4.9 Organic acids (OA)

OA are considered to be any carboxylic acid, including fatty acids and amino acids, which have the general structure R-COOH. Not all of these acids have microbial activity. Those with such activity are short-chain acids (C1-C7), monocarboxylic acids such as formic, acetic, propionic and butyric acids, or acids with a hydroxyl group (usually on carbon a) such as malic, lactic, tartaric and citric acids. They are considered weak acids and are partially dissociated. The OA with the greatest microbial activity are those with a pKa (pH at which half the acid is in dissociated form) between 3 and 5 (DIBNER & BUTTIN, 2002).

The use of organic acids as food additives is not new. They were first used as preservatives to prevent food spoilage and increase the shelf life of perishable ingredients. Specific organic acids have been used to reduce microbial contamination and the spread of food-borne diseases (RICKE, 2003).

The reasons why OA have a nutritional influence on chickens are associated with the deficient production of HCl in diets with a high buffering capacity (high protein and macroelements) and also due to the microbial load acting on the animals (BELLAVER & SCHUERMMAN, 2004).

The toxic effects (direct and indirect) of OA on pathogenic bacteria have not yet been clearly elucidated (RICKE, 2003). However, Mroz (2005) defined some mechanisms of action: 1) the undissociated forms of the acid diffuse through the cell membranes of bacteria, destroying their cytoplasm or inhibiting their growth; 2) dissociation of the acid in the intestine releases H ions^{+} which act as a barrier preventing colonisation by pathogenic bacteria; 3) it reduces gastric pH in complementarity with endogenous HCl; 4) gastric hydrolysis releases H^{+} ions, activating pepsinogen and inhibiting bacterial growth (bactericidal/bacteriostatic effect); 5) supply of an energy substrate/modulator for the development of the intestinal mucosa, improving its absorption capacity; 6) supply of precursors for the synthesis of non-essential amino acids, DNA and lipids necessary for intestinal development; 7) increased blood flow and hypocholesterolaemic effect.

Also according to the same author, after absorption, OA can fulfil various regulatory functions in the growth of the intestinal mucosa, proliferation of epithelial cells, apoptosis and regulation of transcriptional proteins, modulation of gene expression, balance of the acid-base system and energy metabolism.

According to Fascina (2011), OA can also increase the osmotic pressure and, consequently, the pressure on the bacterial cell membrane, causing it to rupture. The absorption of OA in its undissociated form occurs in the intestinal epithelium by passive diffusion.

After ingestion, the antimicrobial activity is most pronounced in the upper GIT, which has a very limited ability to alter the pH of the ingestion. In the ingluvium and proventriculus, OA will reduce the microbial load, being particularly effective against E. coli and other opportunistic acid-intolerant pathogens such as Campylobacter and Salmonella. The consequent reduction in subclinical infections can improve digestibility, reduce the demand for nutrients by gut-associated lymphoid tissue and reduce the production of ammonia and other microbial metabolites (DIBNER & BUTTIN, 2002).

However, acid-tolerant bacteria can survive the pH variations caused by OA. Like antibiotics, bacteria also have different levels of sensitivity to OA. In their undissociated form, acids cannot cross the cell wall of bacteria. The only way to ensure that dissociation takes place in the intestinal lumen is to protect them inside a matrix that has the capacity to pass through the upper part of the GIT without denaturing. Once in the intestine, the matrix is degraded by hepatic and pancreatic enzymes, releasing the OA still in its undissociated form (GAUTHIER, 2002).

In the study carried out by Van Immerseel et al. (2004), microspheres containing acetic, propionic, formic and butyric acids were tested on broilers contaminated with Salmonella Enteritidis. Coated butyric acid was shown to reduce colonisation of the caecum by the bacteria, but had no effect on colonisation of the birds' liver and spleen. Another study by Van Immerseel et al. (2005) compared the efficacy of encapsulated and non-encapsulated butyric acid in specific pathogens free (SPF) chickens and day-old chicks inoculated with Salmonella Enteritidis. The authors found that in SPF chickens, coated butyric acid reduced caecal colonisation three days after infection, while non-encapsulated OA had no effect. In the one-day-old chicks, the treatment receiving encapsulated OA showed a reduction in the number of birds eliminating the bacteria in their faeces, but caecal colonisation remained the same in both groups.

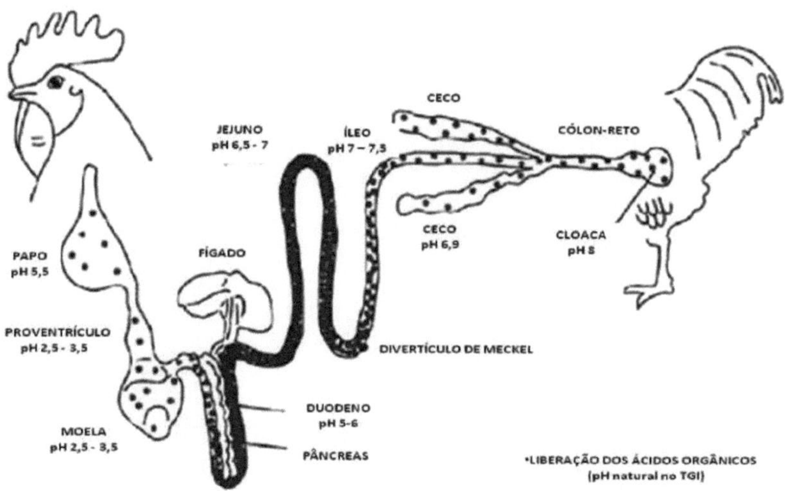

Adapted and redrawn from Riis & Jokobsen, 1969 Hill, 1971, Simon & Versteeg, 1989 and Herpol and Van Grembergen, 1967

FIGURE 02 - Release pattern of encapsulated organic acids in the gastrointestinal tract of chickens

Source: Adapted from GAUTHIER (2002)

Another application of OA is the sanitisation of poultry carcasses. This measure is not intended to cover up hygiene failures that may occur during the rearing and/or slaughter of animals, but rather to complement good production practices in order to reduce pathogens in meat (BELLAVER & SCHUERMMAN, 2002). Mani-Lopéz et al. (2011) stated that the use of OA in the sanitisation of poultry products can prevent outbreaks of salmonellosis in humans.

The lack of consistency in demonstrating the effects of OA is related to uncontrolled variables such as: different dosages and mechanisms of action of the OA used, buffering capacity of dietary ingredients, presence of other antimicrobial compounds, cleanliness of the production environment, variety of intestinal microbiota and the variable analysed. Further research can elucidate the role of these factors and the best way to administer them (DIBNER & BUTTIN, 2002; FRANCO, 2009).

There is a wide variety of OA available for use in broiler diets. The variety and mechanism of action of the OA are important points that influence its activity on the animals' bodies (FRANCO, 2009). The most commonly used OA in poultry farming are formic, acetic, propionic, butyric, lactic, citric and fumaric (LEANDRO et al., 2010).

TABLE 03 - Characteristics of some short-chain fatty acids

AGCC	Specific Effect	Benefits
All AGCC	- pH reduction	• Decreased availability of alkaline cytotoxic compounds • Growth inhibition of pH-sensitive microorganisms
Acetate	• Possible increase in Ca and Mg absorption	• Reduced Ca and Mg excretion

	• Decreased vascular resistance	• Increased blood flow to the colon and liver
Propionate	• Improved colon muscle contraction • Decreased vascular resistance • Stimulation of electrolyte transport through the colon • Growth of colonic epithelial cells	• Facilitates defecation and relieves constipation • Increased blood flow to the colon and liver • Greater absorption of fluids and ions, prevention of diarrhoea. • Improved intestinal absorptive capacity
Butyrate	• Decreased vascular resistance • Colonocyte metabolism • Maintenance of the normal colonocyte phenotype • Stimulation of electrolyte transport through the colon	• Increased blood flow to the colon and liver • Maintenance of mucosal integrity, repair of ulcerative colitis, colonocyte proliferation • Decreased risk of malignant neoplastic formations • Increased absorption of fluids and ions, prevention of diarrhoea

Source: Adapted from TOPPING (1996)

Propionic acid is oily, has a rancid odour and has high antifungal and, to a lesser extent, antibacterial activity. Its high pKa value means that this acid works best at a higher pH (VIOLA, 2006; FRANCO, 2009). Formic acid, on the other hand, is considered a strong acid and its bactericidal action is mainly related to the formate ion, which has a denaturing property on proteins, with good efficiency in controlling microorganisms (MARTINS, 2005). When evaluating the joint action of formic and propionic acids added to the diet of broilers experimentally inoculated with S. enterica serovar Enteritidis, Bassan et al. (2008) found that on the 18th day of the experiment, 40% of the birds that received the OA mixture no longer had the bacteria in their faeces and caecal tonsils.

Lactic acid has good antibacterial activity (DIBNER & BUTTIN, 2002) and is produced both by the lactic fermentation of carbohydrates and sugars such as glucose, lactose and sucrose, and by various bacteria such as Lactobacillus spp., Sporolactobacillus spp., Lactococcus spp., Bacillus spp., Pediococcus spp. and bifidobacteria. Citric acid is a weak acid found in all citrus fruits, known for being a natural antioxidant and having an important function in the Krebs cycle. Acetic acid is a colourless liquid with a penetrating odour, soluble in water, and its impure form is known as vinegar (FASCINA, 2011). This acid is produced by the bacteria Acicodema aceti and Acetobacter through the oxidation of alcohol (VIOLA, 2006).

Using a feed acidified with lactic and acetic acids to feed broilers contaminated with Salmonella sp. and Campylobacter, Heres et al. (2004) observed that the birds fed the acidified feed were less susceptible to Campylobacter infection, but this effect was limited, and there were no inhibitory effects for Salmonella sp. In the study conducted by Rezende et al.
(2008), broiler chickens were given feed contaminated with Enteritidis and Typhimurium serovars and then treated with acetic acid in different concentrations. The researchers found that including the acid in the diet favoured weight gain and feed conversion, but had no effect on reducing the pathogens in the feed.

Fumaric acid has a high dissociation potential and is produced by the degradation of phenylalanine and tyrosine. It also occurs as an intermediate in the urea cycle and in the synthesis of purines (LEHNEN, 2009; SANTOS, 2010). 2-Hydroxy-4-methylthio-butanoic acid (HMTBa) has sulphur in its composition and is converted into methionine in the body (DIBNER & BUTTIN, 2002). Benzoic acid is a weak acid produced in the chemical industry by oxidising toluene or from benzene. This acid is a precursor in the synthesis of many organic substances, and one of its best-known derivatives is 2-acetylsalicylic acid (FASCINA, 2011).

In the study by Rocha et al. (2011), a mixture of acids (benzoic, fumaric and HMTBa) was used in the feed of broilers inoculated with nalidixic acid-resistant Salmonella Typhimurium via the gut and via the feed. It was observed that the birds inoculated with the bacteria and treated with the OA, regardless of the route, showed better results in terms of average weight, weight gain, feed conversion and greater duodenal villus height.

The use of OA in the diet and drinking water has shown promising results in modulating the intestinal microbiota. Nava et al. (2009), using molecular identification techniques to characterise the intestinal microbial population after supplementation of different OA mixtures in broiler feed, observed that the mixture of formic, propionic and HMTBa acids affected the intestinal microbiota, generating more homogeneous populations and increasing colonisation by Lactobacillus spp. in the poultry ileum.

In the study carried out by Pickler et al. (2012), which analysed the effects of a commercial additive containing different mixtures of OA on broilers inoculated with the Enteritidis and Minnesota serovars, it was observed that the inclusion of OA in feed and drinking water reduced the presence of Salmonella in the poultry droppings and cecum excretion, and was more effective for the Enteritidis serovar than the Minnesota serovar.

Butyric acid is obtained through the fermentation of carbohydrates in the rumen of polygastrics and the colon of omnivores (KIEN et al., 2000). This OA is known to influence the growth of intestinal mucosal cells and improve the retention of calcium and phosphorus in the diet (DIBNER & BUTTIN, 2002). When analysing the effects of butyric acid inoculation on embryonated eggs, Leandro et al. (2010) observed that chicks from eggs treated with butyrate showed an increase in intestinal biometry when compared to the control group (without the acid), but there was no improvement in the birds' performance (up to 10 days of age). Testing the interaction between butyric and lactic acids, Salazar et al. (2008) found that the use of butyric acid during the initial phase and the combination of butyric and lactic acid during the growth phase improved broiler performance results.

In a study by Viola & Vieira (2007), the performance and intestinal morphology of broilers fed diets containing antibiotics and different mixtures of organic acids were evaluated. The researchers found that the zootechnical performance and intestinal morphology of the animals given the OA were similar to those given antibiotics in the diet. Also using a feed additive containing a mixture of different OA in the diet of broilers inoculated with Salmonella Enteritidis and Eimeria tenella, Calaça (2009) observed that the inclusion of OA reduced the frequencies of isolation of the Enteridis serovar in the spleen and caecal tonsils of the birds, even when challenged concomitantly with E. tenella.

OA are promising alternatives to the use of AMD in animal production and the application of the associated form (free acids + protected acids) seems to be the best way to be used in animal feed. Further studies are needed to define the best combinations and dosages of acids (FRANCO, 2009).

4.10 Phytogenic

Phytogenic additives are plant-derived compounds that are added to animal diets in order to improve the productivity and quality of the products produced by these animals. This class of additives has recently gained greater interest, causing a significant increase in publications since 2000 (WINDISCH et al., 2007). The most important factor contributing to the emergence of this interest in the use of plants in animal production is the rigour of legislation surrounding conventional additives such as antibiotics, anticoccidials and anthelmintics (GREATHEAD, 2003).

Other terms are used to classify the wide variety of phytogenic compounds, mainly referring to origin or processing, such as herbs (flowering, non-persistent plants), spices (herbs with an intense smell and flavour, commonly used in cooking), essential oils (lipophilic volatile compounds), oleoresins (extracts obtained by non-aqueous solvents). Within the group of phytogenic additives, the content of active substances can vary widely depending on the part of the plant used (seed, leaf, root, bark), harvest season, geographical origin and extraction technique (WINDISCH et al., 2007). The difference between plant extracts (VE) and essential oils (EO) is the extraction method. EOs are only obtained through steam extraction (OETTING, 2005).

Phytogenic additives are commonly used in animal diets to improve palatability and production performance. However, studies demonstrating the effects of including phytogenic additives on palatability are very scarce. What has been researched most is their influence on feed consumption and animal weight gain

(COSTA, 2009).

The active principles of plants are classified according to their physical, chemical and biological properties. These principles are not found in plants in their pure state, but in complex form, the components of which reinforce their action on the organism (OETTING, 2005).

Although the mechanisms of action of phytogenic additives have not been fully elucidated, Oetting (2005) cites some hypotheses: 1) modulation of the intestinal microbiota through their antimicrobial activity; 2) antioxidant activity; 3) stimulation of enzymatic activity and nutrient absorption; 4) morphological changes in the intestinal epithelium, organ morphometry and reduction in ammonia production.

The antimicrobial properties of phytogenics are determined by their physicochemical characteristics, such as pH, solubility, pKa and polarity (NEGI et al., 2012). These compounds have a dose-dependent bactericidal and bacteriostatic action on viruses, bacteria, fungi and protozoa (COSTA, 2009). In an evaluation of the antimicrobial effects of phytogenics, Dorman & Deans (2000) defined a descending order for the efficiency of the compounds: thymol, carvracol, a-terpineol, terpinen-4-ol, eugenol, (±)-linalool, (-)-thujone, õ-3-carene, cis-hex-3-na-1-ol, geranyl acetate, (cis + *trans)* citral, nerol, geraniol, menthone, 0-pinene, R(+) limonene, a-pinene, a-terpinene, borneol, (+)-sabinene, Y-terpinene, citronella, 1,8-cineol, bornyl acetate, carvracol methyl ether, myrcene, 0-caryophyllene, a-bisabolol, a-felandrene, a-humulene, 0-bocimeme, aromadrendene, p-cymene.

Due to the wide variety of chemical compounds, the antimicrobial capacity of EOs is not attributed to just one specific mechanism, but to several targets within the cell. These targets are often not reached separately; some are affected as a result of another target being reached (BURT, 2004).

An important characteristic of EOs is their hydrophobicity, which allows them to interact with the bacterial cell membrane. By disrupting the cellular structure of microorganisms, their contents leak out and ATPase activity is inhibited (BURT, 2004). Gram negative bacteria have a hydrophilic cell wall which creates a physical barrier to the action of EOs, making these microorganisms resistant (COSTA, 2009).

According to Kamel (2001), an important mechanism of action of certain EVs may be their ability to influence bacterial cell surface characteristics, such as hydrophobicity, and consequently alter their virulence properties. This has implications for the intestinal health of animals, since the adhesion of pathogens to host cells is strongly influenced by the hydrophobicity of the microbial cell surface.

According to Huyghebaert (2003), each plant species has a different intensity of antimicrobial activity. Ginger and chilli are considered weak, oregano, rosemary, thyme, cumin, coriander and sage are medium and cloves, mustard, cinnamon and garlic have high activity against microorganisms.

Another possible contribution of phytogenic products in the control of pathogens is the stimulation of intestinal mucus production, which reduces the adherence of these bacteria to the intestinal mucosa (WINDISCH et al., 2007).

EOs degrade the bacterial cell wall, causing damage to the cytoplasmic membrane and membrane proteins, outflow of cell contents, coagulation of the cytoplasm and depletion of the proton motive force, as shown in Figure 03.

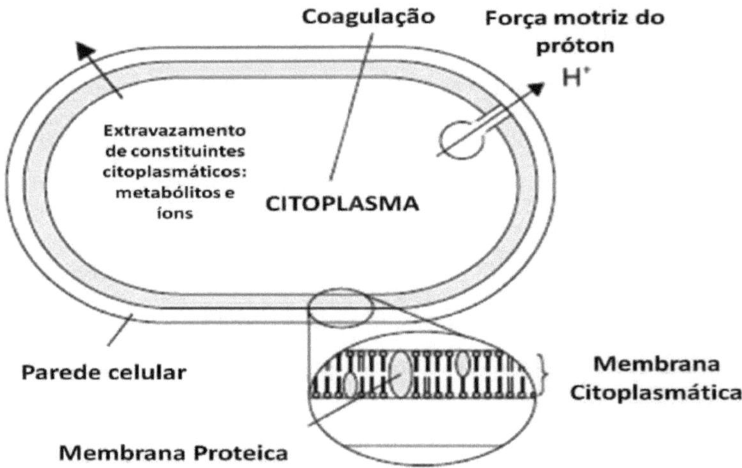

FIGURE 03 - Mechanisms of action and localisation of the sites of action of essential oil components

Source: Adapted from BURT (2004).

Silvàn et al. (2012) analysed the antibacterial activity of grape seed extract against different Campylobacter samples. The study showed a strong inhibitory capacity for the agent tested. Analysis of the antimicrobial activity showed that phenolic acids, catechins and proanthocyanidins were the main factors responsible for this behaviour.

In the study carried out by Wiest et al. (2009), the intensity of bacterial inhibition activity and the intensity of bacterial inactivation activity in vitro against Salmonella sp. of 86 medicinal or spicy plants found in the Porto Alegre - RS region were checked. Of the plants tested, 50 showed some selective activity against the bacteria. Leek, garlic, macela, chilli pepper, yerba mate, oregano, sage and chinchilla stood out for their antimicrobial capacity.

Evaluating three levels of inclusion of a mixture of oregano, aniseed and citrus EOs on the composition of the caecal microbiota of broiler chickens, Mountzouris et al. (2011) found that there was an increase in the populations of Lactobacillus, Bifidobacterium and Gram-positive cocci and a reduction in intestinal colonisation by faecal coliforms in the birds that received the EOs via feed. Similarly, Agostini et al. (2012) analysed the effects of different levels of clove EO in broiler feed on the intestinal microbiota. The authors noted that the inclusion of the phytogenic did not affect bacteria from the Enterobacteriaceae family, but the Lactobacillus population increased compared to the control treatment. Kirkpinar et al. (2011), using oregano and garlic EOs in feed, observed that the counts of Lactobacillus spp. and Streptococcus were unchanged, but the number of clostridia was reduced in the birds given oregano alone and oregano combined with garlic.

According to Mellor (2000), some plants can stimulate efficient digestion by increasing the secretion of salivary glands and gastric and pancreatic juices. In addition to increased enzyme secretion, changes in organ morphometry, oronasal sensory stimulation and control of pathogenic microorganisms are possible hypotheses to justify this increase in digestibility (UTIYAMA, 2004; BRENES & ROURA, 2010).

In their study, Rizzo et al. (2010) evaluated the effects of including EOs compared to an antibiotic (avilamycin) on the performance of broiler chickens. The

EOs used were cinnamon, clove, thyme, pepper, oregano, eucalyptus, cinnamon, boldo-do-chile and fenugreek in different combinations and concentrations. The authors concluded that the addition of these phytogenics had no significant effect on performance when compared to the diet without additives and the diet with antibiotics. The authors also emphasised that due to the absence of a microbiological challenge and the high quality of the diet, the possible effects of adding EOs may not have been detected. Barreto et al. (2008) also used different types of EOs in feed and evaluated their effects on broiler performance. Clove, red pepper, oregano and cinnamon extracts were used, as well as an antibiotic (avilamycin), as a comparative. The researchers did not observe any effect of the plant extracts on the birds' performance.

Gastrointestinal morphological changes suggest the beneficial effects of phytogenics, but there are no consistent reports in the available literature (COSTA, 2009). Evaluating the effects of including red mastic oil in broiler rations, Silva et al. (2011) found that the animals treated with the phytogenic had a higher villus:crypt ratio compared to the treatment that did not receive any additive.

Another way of assessing the effects of phytogenics is by analysing organ biometrics (COSTA, 2009). Fascina (2011) carried out a study in which the inclusion of phytogenics (turmeric, citrus and grape seed extracts + cinnamon EO, boldo-do-chile leaves and fenugreek seeds), organic acids (lactic, benzoic, formic, citric and acetic acids) and antibiotics (avilamycin and monensin sodium) was assessed in broiler organ biometry. The results showed that the birds supplemented with the phytogenics had greater pancreas weight (21 days) and greater length of the small and large intestines (42 days), compared to the treatments that received the acidifiers and antibiotics. However, Kirkpinar et al. (2011) found no significant differences in the biometry of bird organs when using oregano and garlic alone or in combination in the diet.

The amount of ammonia in the intestine is directly related to the microbiota. Its toxicity increases cell turnover in the intestinal epithelium, causing greater energy expenditure for the animal. Modulating the microbiota can reduce ammonia production and consequently protect the integrity of the mucosa, improving its absorptive capacity

(UTIYAMA, 2004). Cypriano et al. (2009) included a mixture of thyme EO, fennel EO and EVs of pepper, gentian and quillaia in the feed offered to broiler chickens and found that there was an improvement in performance and a reduction in the ammonia content in the house in the treatment that received the phytogenics in the feed.

Plants and their bioactive compounds can also increase the immune function of animals. According to various reports, there have been anti-inflammatory effects, improvement in humoral and cellular immunity and modulation of immune pathways, specific receptors, enzymes and immune molecules (DURMIC & BLACHE, 2012). In the study carried out by Agostini et al. (2012), different levels of clove were included in the diet of broiler chickens. The results showed that the inclusion of cloves increased the number of lymphocytes and the cell density of the lamina propria of the birds' intestines. However, Cardoso et al. (2012) observed a significant decrease in monocytes when they added black pepper to poultry feed.

The variation in the efficiency of EOs in animal production is mainly due to the following factors: feed composition (less digestible ingredients), dietary intake level, hygiene standards and environmental conditions. Other factors that could influence the results of experiments carried out in vivo include: the time and method of harvesting, the ripeness of the plant, the method of preservation, the duration of storage and the possible synergistic or antagonistic effect of bioactive compounds (BRENE & ROURA, 2011).

CHAPTER 6

FINAL CONSIDERATIONS

The presence of Salmonella in Brazilian poultry is an obstacle to achieving a desirable level of health on farms and consequently in the food products that come from this sector. The wide variety of sources of infection for broiler chickens and the presence of recontamination and cross-contamination between them, means that Salmonella perpetuates itself in the production environment, even if it is carefully controlled.

Antibiotics and chemotherapy drugs have long been one of the main tools for controlling Salmonella in the production environment. However, with the ban on the use of these drugs in animal production, the competitiveness of this sector is under threat. Finding substitutes for antibiotics has become of fundamental importance for maintaining the productivity and safety of food of animal origin.

Within this context, alternative feed additives have gained prominence. The various types of prebiotics, probiotics, symbiotics, organic acids and phytogenics have been studied in an effort to discover the best additive and/or combination of additives that can be used as growth modulators.

Further research is needed to determine important aspects such as: best dose-response, effects of combining additives, toxicity, effectiveness on animal performance, cost-benefit and possible implications for the environment.

REFERENCES

1. AARESTRUP, F. M.; SEYFARTH, A. M.; EMBORG, H. D.; PEDERSEN, K.; HENDRIKSEN, R. S.; BAGER, F. Effect of abolishment of the use of antimicrobial agents for growth promotion on occurrence of antimicrobial resistance in faecal enterococci from food animals in Denmark. Antimicrobial Agents and Chemotherapy, Washington, v. 45, n. 7, p. 2054-2059, 2001.

2. ALBINO, L. F. T., FERES, F. A., DIONIZIO, M. A., ROSTAGNO, H. S., JÚNIOR, J. G. V., CARVALHO, D. C. O., GOMES, P. C., COSTA, C. H. R. Use of prebiotics based on mannan oligosaccharides in broiler rations. Revista Brasileira de Zootecnia, Viçosa, v. 3, n. 35, p. 742-749, 2006.

3. AGOSTINI, P. S.; SOLÀ-ORIOL, D.; NOFRARÍAS, M.; BARROETA, A. C.; GASA, J.; MANZANILLA, E. G. Role of in-feed clove supplementation on growth performance, intestinal microbiology and morphology in broiler chicken. Livestock Science, Foulum, v. 147, p. 113-118, 2012.

4. ANDRADE, M. A.; MESQUITA, A. J.; STRINGHINI, J. H.; BRITO, L. A. B.; CHAVES, L. S.; MATTOS, M. S. Clinical and anatomo-pathological aspects of broiler chicks from eggs experimentally inoculated with Salmonella Enteritidis phage 4. Ciência Animal Brasileira, Goiânia, v. 10, n. 3, p. 909-917, 2009.

5. ANDREATTI FILHO, R. L. Avian paratyphoid. In: ANDREATTI FILHO, R. L. Avian Health and Diseases, Ed. Roca, São Paulo, 2007.

6. ANDREATTI FILHO, R. L.; LIMA, E. T.; MENCONI, A.; ROCHA, T. S.; GONÇALVES, G. A. M. Detection of Salmonella spp. in trawl feeds from poultry farms. Veterinária e Zootecnia, São Paulo, v. 16, n. 1, 2009.

7. ARAÚJO, J. C.; SILVA, J. H. V.; AMÂNCIO, A. L. L.; LIMA, M. R., LIMA, C. B. Use of additives in poultry feed. Acta Veterinária Brasílica, Mossoró, v.1, n. 3, p. 69-77, 2007.

8. AURELI, P.; CAPURSO, L.; CASTELLAZZI, A. M.; CLERICI, M.; GIOVANNINI, M.; MORELLI, L.; POLI, A.; PREGLIASCO, F.; SALVINI, F.; ZUCCOTTI, G. V. Probiotics and health: an evidence-based review. Pharmacological Research, Madrid, v. 63, n. 5, p. 366-376, 2011.

9. AWAD, W.; GHAREEB, K.; BOHM, J. Intestinal structure and function of broiler chickens on diets supplemented with a synbiotic containing Enterococcus faecium and oligosaccharides. International Journal of Molecular Science, Basel, v. 9, n. 11, p. 2205-2216, 2008.

10. BASSAN, J. D. L.; FLÔRES, M. L.; ANTONIAZZI, T.; BIANCHI, E.; KUTTEL, J.; TRINDADE, M. M. Control of Salmonella Enteritidis infection in broilers with organic acids and mannan oligosaccharides. Ciência Rural, Santa Maria, v. 38, n. 7, p. 1961-1965, 2008.

11. BARRETO, M. R. S.; MENTEN, J. F. M.; RACANICCI, A. M. C.; PEREIRA, P. W. Z.; RIZZO, P. V. Plant extracts used as growth promoters in broilers, Brazilian Journal of Poultry Science, Piracicaba, v. 10, n. 2, p. 109-115, 2008.

12. BAURHOO, B.; LETELLIER, A.; ZHAO, X.; RUIZ-FERIA, C. A. Cecal populations of lactobacilli and bifidobacteria and Escherichia coli populations after in vivo Escherichia coli challenge in birds fed diets with purified lignin or mannanoligosaccharides. Poultry Science, Champaign, v. 86, n. 12, p. 2509-2516, 2007.

13. BELLAVER, C.; SCHEUERMANN, G. Applications of organic acids in poultry production. Lecture presented at the AVISUI 2004 Conference. Florianópolis, SC, 2004.

14. BERCHIERI JÚNIOR, A.; FREITAS NETO, O. C. Salmonellosis. In: BERCHIERI JÚNIOR, A.; SILVA, E. N.; DI FÁBIO, J.; SESTI, L.; ZUANAZE, M. A. F. Poultry diseases, 2ª edition, Ed. FACTA, Campinas, 2009.

15. BONI, H. F. K.; CARRIJO, A. S.; FASCINA, V. B. Occurrence of Salmonella spp. in poultry houses and broiler slaughterhouses in the central region of Mato Grosso do Sul. Revista Brasileira de Saúde e Produção Animal, Salvador, v. 12, n. 1, p. 84-95, 2011.

16. BORSOI, A.; MORAES, H. L. S; SALLE, C. T. P.; NASCIMENTO, V. P. Most probable number of Salmonella isolated from chilled chicken carcasses. Ciência Rural, Santa Maria, v. 40, n. 11, p. 2338-2342, 2010.

17. BRAZIL. Health Surveillance Secretariat/UHA/CGDT. Epidemiological data - ATDs from 2000-2011. Ministry of Health, 2012.

18. BRAZIL. Ministry of Agriculture, Livestock and Supply. Normative Instruction No. 15, of 26 May 2009, Regulating the registration of establishments and products intended for animal feed. Brasília: Ministry of Agriculture, Livestock and Supply, 2009.

19. BRENES, A.; ROURA, E. Essential oils in poultry nutrition: main effects and modes of action. Animal Feed Science and Technology, Amsterdam, v. 158, p. 1-14, 2010.

20. BRISBIN, J. T.; GONG, J.; SHARIF, S. Interactions between commensal bacteria and the gut-associated immune system of the chicken. Animal Health Research Reviews, Canada, v. 9, n. 1, p. 101-110, 2008.

21. BURT, S. Essential oils: their antibacterial properties and potential applications in foods--a review. International Journal of Food Microbiology, Torino, v. 94, n. 3, p. 223-253, 2004.

22. CALAÇA, G. M. Organic acids in the control of Salmonella Enteritidis in broilers experimentally challenged with Salmonella Enteritidis and Eimeria tenella. 2009. 70 f. Dissertation (Master's in Animal Health) - Veterinary and Zootechnical School, Federal University of Goiás, Goiânia.

23. CALLAWAY, T. R.; EDRINGTON, T. S.; ANDERSON, R. C.; HARVEY, R. B.; GENOVESE, K. J.; KENNEDY, C. N.; VENN, D. W.; NISBET, D. J. Probiotics, prebiotics and competitive exclusion for prophylaxis against bacterial disease.

Animal Health Research Reviews, Canada, v. 9, n. 2, p. 217-225, 2008.

24. CARAMORI JÚNIOR, J. G.; ROÇA, R. L.; FRAGA, A. L.; VIEITES, F. M.; MORCELLI, L.; GONÇALVES, M. A. Effect of Symbiotics in the initial ration of broiler chickens on performance, carcass and meat quality. Acta Scientiarum Animal Science, Maringá, v. 30, n. 1, p. 17-23, 2008.

25. CARDOSO, T. G.; CARVALHO, V. M. Toxinfecção alimentar por Salmonella spp. Revista do Instituto de Ciências da Saúde, São Paulo, v. 24, n. 2, p. 95-101, 2006.

26. CARDOSO, A. L. S. P.; TESSARI, E. N. C. Salmonella in food safety. Arquivo do Instituto Biológico, Descalvado, v. 70, n.1, p. 1113, 2008.

27. CARDOSO, V. S.; LIMA, C. A. R.; LIMA, M. E. F.; DORNELES, L. E. G.; DANELLI, M. G. M. Piperine as a phytogenic additive in broiler diets.

Pesquisa Agropecuária Brasileira, Brasília, v. 47, n. 4, p. 489-496, 2012.

28. CARVALHO, A. C. B. F.; FLORIOTO, J. F.; SCHOCKEN-ITURRINO, R. B. Campylobacter and Salmonella in faeces and in different types of poultry litter. ARS Veterinária, v.17, n. 3, p. 201-206, 2001.

29. CARVALHO, A. C. F. B.; CORTEZ, A. L. L. Salmonella sp. in carcasses, mechanically separated meat, sausages and commercial chicken cuts. Ciência Rural, Santa Maria, v. 35, n. 6, p. 1465-1468, 2005.

30. CENTER FOR DISEASE CONTROL, Salmonella Surveillance: Annual Summary, 2006. Atlanta, Georgia: United States Department of Health and Human Services, CDC, 2008.

31. CENTER FOR DISEASE CONTROL, National Salmonella Surveillance Overview. Atlanta, Georgia: United States Department of Health and Human Service, CDC, 2011.

32. CENTER FOR DISEASE CONTROL, Multistate Outbreak of Salmonella Braenderup Infections Associated with Mangoes (Final Update). Atlanta, Georgia: United States Department of Health and Human Service, CDC, 2012. Available at: http://www.cdc.gov/salmonella/braenderup-08-12/

33. CENTER FOR DISEASE CONTROL, Multistate Outbreak of Human Salmonella Infections Linked to Live Poultry in Backyard Flocks (Final Update). Atlanta, Georgia: United States Department of Health and Human Service, CDC, 2012. Available at: http://www.cdc.gov/salmonella/live-poultry-05-12/index.html

34. CHERNAKI-LEFFER, A. M.; BIESDORF, S. M.; ALMEIDA, L. M.; LEFFER, E. V. B.; VIGNE, F. Isolation of enterobacteria from Alphitobius diaperinus in poultry litter in western Paraná State, Brazil. Revista Brasileira de Ciência Avícola, Campinas, v. 4, n. 3, p. 243-247, 2002.

35. CHINIVASAGAM, H. N.; TRAN, T.; BLACKALL, P. J. Impact of the Australian litter re-use practice on Salmonella in the broiler farming environment. Food Research International, Barking, v. 45, p. 891-896, 2012.

36. CORCIONIVOSCHI, N., DRINCEANU, D., POP, I. M., STACK, D., STEF, L., JULEAN, C., BOURKE, B. The effects of probiotics on animal health.

Journal of Animal Science and Biotechnologies, London, v.43, n.1, p. 35-41.

37. CORRIGAN, A.; HORGAN, K.; CLIPSON, N.; MURPHY, R. A. Effect of dietary supplementation with a Saccharomyces cerevisiae mannan oligosaccharide on the bacterial community structure of broiler caecal contents. Applied and Environmental Microbiology, Washington, v. 77, n. 18, p. 6653-6662, 2011.

38. COSTA, L. B. Phytogenic additives and sodium butyrate as potential growth promoters for newly weaned piglets. 2009. 96 f. Thesis (Doctorate in Animal and Pasture Science) - Escola Superior de Agronomia "Luiz de Queiroz" - Universidade de São Paulo, Piracicaba.

39. COX , N. A., BERRANGE, M. E., CASON, J. A. Salmonella penetration of egg shells and proliferation in broiler hatching eggs. Poultry Science, Champaign, v. 79, n.11, p.1571-1574, 2000.

40. CYPRIANO, L.; PICCINI, I.; FILHO, L. B. P.; WENDLER, K. R. Use of phytogenic additives in broiler diets - 1st cycle. 27ª FACTA Conference on Poultry Science and Technology. Porto Alegre, RS. Proceedings...Porto Alegre, 2009, CD ROOM.

41. DIBNER, J. J.; RICHARDS, J. D. Antibiotic growth promoters in agriculture: history and mode of action. Poultry Science, Champaign, v. 84, n. 4, p. 634-643, 2005.

42. DIBNER, J. J., BUTTIN, P. Use of organic acids as a model to study the impact of gut microflora on nutritionand metabolism. The Journal of Applied Poutry Research, Champaign, v. 11, p. 453-463, 2002.

43. DIONÍSIO, M. A.; BERTECHINI, A. G.; KATO, R. K.; TEIXEIRA, A. S. Prebiotics as growth promoters for broilers - Performance and carcass yield. Ciência e Agrotecnologia, Lavras, Special Ed., p. 1580-1587, 2002.

44. DORMAN, H. J. D., DEANS, S. G. Antimicrobial agents from plants: antibacterial activity of plant volatile oils. Journal of Applied Microbiology, Oxford, v. 88, p. 308-319, 2000.

45. DONALSON, L. M.; KIM, W. K.; CHALOVA, V. I.; HERRERA, P.; WOODWARD, C. L.; MCREYNOLDS, J. L.; KUBENA, L. F.; NISBET, D. J.; RICKE, S. C. In vitro anaerobic incubation of Salmonella enterica

serotype Typhimurium and laying hen caecal bacteria in poultry feed substrates and a fructooligosaccharide prebiotic. Anaerobe, Iowa, v. 13, n. 5-6, p. 208-214, 2007.

46. DURMIC, Z.; BLACHE, D. Bioactive plants and plant products: effects on animal function, health and welfare, Animal Feed Science and Technology, Amsterdam, v. 176, p. 150-162, 2012.

47. FAO/OIE/WHO. Expert Workshop on Non-Human Antimicrobial Usage and Antimicrobial Resistance: Scientific assessment. Geneva, 2003. http://www.who.int/foodsafety/micro/meetings/nov2003/en/.

48. FARIA FILHO, D. E.; TORRES, K. A. A.; FARIA, D. E.; CAMPOS, D. M. B; ROSA, P. S. Probiotics for broiler chickens in Brazil: systematic review and meta-analysis. Brazilian Journal of Poultry Science, Jaboticabal, v. 8, n. 2, p. 89-98, 2006.

49. FASCINA, V. B. Phytogenic additives and organic acids in broiler diets. 2011.175 f. Thesis (Doctorate in Animal Nutrition and Production) - Universidade Estadual Paulista, Botucatu.

50. FEARNLEY, E.; RAUPACH, J.; LAGALA, F.; CAMERON, S. Salmonella in chicken meat, eggs and humans; Adelaide, South Australia, 2008. International Journal of Food Microbiology, Amsterdam, v. 146, p. 219-227, 2011.

51. FERREIRA, E. O.; CAMPOS, L. C. Salmonella. In: TRABULSI, L. R.; ALTERTHUM, F. Microbiologia, 5ª edition. Ed. Atheneu, São Paulo, 2008.

52. FIORENTIN, L. Reuse of litter in broiler rearing and the bacteriological implications for human and animal health. Concórdia: Embrapa Swine and Poultry, 2005. 23p. (Embrapa Swine and Poultry. Documents, 94).

53. FLACHOWSKY, G. Book review - Animal Feed Contamination-Effects on Livestock and Food Safety, FINK-GREMMELS J. (Ed.), Woodhead Publishing Series in Food Science, Technology and Nutrition, Vol. 215 WP - Woodhead Publishing Limited, Oxford/Cambridge/Philadelphia/New Delhi (2012). 672 p, 2012.

54. FLEMMING, J. S., Use of yeasts, probiotics and mannan oligosaccharides (MOS) in broiler feed.

2005. 111 f. Thesis (Doctorate in Food Technology) - Federal University of Paraná, Curitiba.

55. FRANCO, L. G. Organic acids as an alternative to the use of performance-enhancing antimicrobials in broiler chickens. 2009. 74 f. Dissertation (Master's Degree in Animal Quality and Productivity) - Faculty of Animal Science and Food Engineering, University of São Paulo, Pirassununga.

56. FREITAS NETO, O. C.; PENHA FILHO, R. A. C.; BARROW, P.; BERCHIERI JÚNIOR, A. Sources of humannon-typhoid salmonellosis: a review. Brazilian Journal of Poultry Science, Campinas, v. 12, n. 1, p. 01-11, 2010.

57. FURLAN, R. L., MACARI, M., LUQUETTI, B. C. How to evaluate the effects of using prebiotics, probiotics and competitive exclusion flora. In: 5th Technical Symposium on Incubation, Broiler Breeding and Nutrition, 2004, Balneário Camboriú. Proceedings...Santa Catarina, p. 6-26, 2004.

58. GAGGIA, F.; MATTARELLI, P.; BIAVATI, B. Probiotics and prebiotics in animal feeding for safe food production. International Journal of Food Microbiology, Torino, v. 141 Suppl 1, n. p. S15-28, 2010.

59. GAMBIRAGI, A. P. O. M.; SALLES, R. P. R.; AGUIAR FILHO, J. L.; OLIVEIRA, W. F.; MACIEL, W. C.; ROMÃO, J. M.; TEIXEIRA, R. S. C. Salmonella sp. in one-day-old broilers from the metropolitan region of Fortaleza-CE. Acta Scientiae Veterinariae, Porto Alegre, v. 31, n. 3, p. 149-153, 2003.

60. GAUTHIER, R. Intestinal Health: Key to Productivity (The Case of Organic Acids). In: IASA Poultry Scientific Congress, XXVII ANECA-WPDC Convention. Puerto Vallarta, Jal. Mexico, 2002. *Electronic* proceedings... [on line] Available at: http://www.engormix.com/MA- avicultura/nutricion/articulos/salud-intestinal-clave-productividad- t518/p0.htm

61. GIBSON, G. R.; ROBERFROID, M. B. Dietary modulation of the human colonic microbiota: Introducing the concept of prebiotics. *The Journal of Nutrition*, Amsterdam, v. 125, p. 1401-1412, 1995.

62. GREATHEAD, H. Plants and plant extracts for improving animal productivity. *Proceedings of the Nutrition Society,* Netherlands, v. 62, n. 2, p. 279-290, 2003.

63. HALL, V. L. M.; MARTIN, J. G. P.; CANDEIAS, J. M. G.; CARDOSO, K. F. G.; SILVA, M. G.; RALL, R.; ARAÚJO JÚNIOR, J. P. Salmonella research and sanitary conditions of chickens and sausages sold in the city of Botucatu. Brazilian

Journal of Veterinary Research and Animal Science, São Paulo, v. 46, n. 3, p. 167-174, 2009.

64. HERES, L.; ENGEL, B.; URLINGS, H. A.; WAGENAAR, J. A.; VAN KNAPEN, F. Effect of acidified feed on susceptibility of broiler chickens to intestinal infection by Campylobacter and Salmonella. Veterinary Microbiology, Geneva, v. 99, n. 3-4, p. 259-267, 2004.

65. HOLT, P. S.; GEDEN, C. J.; MOORE, R. W.; GAST, R. K. Isolation of Salmonella enterica serovar Enteritidis from houseflies (Musca domestica) found in rooms containing Salmonella serovar Enteritidis-challenged hens. Applied and Environmental Microbiology, Washington, v. 73, n. 19, 2007.

66. HOOGE, D. M., Meta-analysis of broiler chicken pen trials evaluating dietary mannan oligosaccharide, 1993-2003. International Journal of Poultry Science, Faisalabad, n. 3, v.3, p. 163-174, 2004.

67. HUGHES, L. A.; SHOPLAND, S.; WIGLEY, P.; BRANDON, H.; LEATHERBARROW, H.; WILLIAN, N. J.; BENNETT, M.; PINNA, E.; LAWSON, B.; CUNNINGHAM, A. A.; CHANTREY, J. Characterisation of Salmonella enterica serotype Typhimurium isolates from wild birds in northern England from 2005-2006. BMC Veterinary Research, v. 4, n. 4, 2008.

68. HUME, M. E. Historic perspective: prebiotics, probiotics, and other alternatives to antibiotics. Poultry Science, Champaign, v. 90, n. 11, p. 2663-2669, 2011.

69. HUYGHEBAERT, G. Replacement of antibiotics in poultry. In: EASTERN NUTRITION CONFERENCE, 2003. Quebec City. Proceedings... Quebec City, p.1-23, 2003.

70. HUYGHEBAERT, G.; DUCATELLE, R.; VAN IMMERSEEL, F. An update on alternatives to antimicrobial growth promoters for broilers. The Veterinary Journal, v. 187, n. 2, p. 182-188, 2011.

71. JONES, F. T.; RICKE, S. C. Observations on the history of the development of antimicrobials and their use in poultry feeds. Poultry Science, Champaign, v. 82, n. 4, p. 613-617, 2003.

72. KAMEL, C. Natural plant extracts: Classical remedies bring modern animal production solutions. Cahiers Options Méditerranéennes, Zaragoza, v. 54, p. 31-38, 2001.

73. KAUR, I. P.; CHOPRA, K.; SAINI, A. Probiotics: potential pharmaceutical applications. European Journal of Pharmaceutical Sciences, Jarfalla v. 15, n. 1, p. 1-9, 2002.

74. KIEN, L. K.; CHANG, J. C.; COOPER, J. R. Butyric acid is synthesised by piglets. American Society for Nutritional Sciences, New York, v. 3, n. p. 234-237, 2000.

75. KIM, A.; LEE, Y. J.; KANG, M. S.; KWAG, S. I.; CHO, J. K. Disseminationand tracking of Salmonella spp. in integrated broiler operation. Journal of Veterinary Science, Suwon, v. 8, n. 2, p. 155-161, 2007.

76. KIM, G. B.; SEO, Y. M.; KIM, S. H.; PAIK, I. K. Effect of dietary prebiotic supplementation on the performance, intestinal microflora and immune response of broilers. Poultry Science, Champaign, v. 90, p. 75-82, 2011.

77. KIRKPINAR, F.; BORA UNLU, H.; OZDEMIR, G. Effects of oregano and garlic essential oils on performance, carcase, organ and blood characteristics and intestinal microflora of broilers, Livestock Science, Foulum, v. 137, p. 219-225, 2011.

78. KOTTWITZ, L. B. M.; OLIVEIRA, T. C. R. M.; ALCOCER, I.; FARAH, S. M. S. S.; ABRAHÃO, W. S. M.; RODRIGUES, D. P. Epidemiological evaluation of salmonellosis outbreaks between 1999 and 2008 in the state of Paraná, Brazil. Acta Scientiarum. Health Science, Maringá, v. 32, n. 1, p. 09-15, 2010.

79. LEANDRO, N. S. M., OLIVEIRA, A. S. C., CAFÉ, M. B., GONZALES, E., STRINGHINI, J. H., CARVALHO, F. B., ANDRADE, M. A. Effect of prebiotics and in ovo butyric acid on performance, digestibility of feed nutrients and gastrointestinal tract biometry of chicks submitted to fasting. Ciência Animal Brasileira, Goiânia, v. 11, n. 4, p. 806-816, 2010.

80. LEHNEN, C. R. Addition of fumaric acid in diets prepared with maize wet grain silage: conservation of diets, performance of sows and litters. 2009. 87 f. Dissertation (Master

in Animal Production) - Centre for Rural Sciences, Federal University of Santa Maria, Santa Maria.

81. LUCCA, W.; CECCHIN, R.; TIMBOLA, E.; GRADIN, J.; LUCCA, M. S. Effect of different chemical treatments on poultry litter. Revista Agroambiental, Pouso Alegre, v. 4, n. 1, p. 25-31, 2012.

82. MANI-LÓPEZ, E., GARCIA, H. S., LÓPEZ-MALO, A. Organic acids as antimicrobial to control Salmonella in meat and poultry products. Food Research International, Toronto, v. 45, p. 713-721, 2012.

83. MACIOROWSKI, K. G.; HERRERA, P.; JONES, F. T.; PILLAI, S. D.; RICKE, S. C.Effects on poultry and livestock of feed contamination with bacteria and fungi . Animal Feed Science and Technology, Amsterdam v. 133, p. 109-136, 2007.

84. MAJOWICZ, S. E.; MUSTO, J.; SCALLAN, E.; ANGULO, F. J.; KIRK, M.; O'BRIEN, S. J.; JONES, T. F.; FAZIL, A.; HOESKTRA, R. M. The global burden of nonthyphoidal *Salmonella* gastroenterits Clinicai Infectious Diseases, Chicago, v. 50, p. 882-889, 2010.

85. MARIN, C.; BALASCH, S.; VEGA, S.; LAINEZ, M. Sources of Salmonella contamination during broiler production in Eastern Spain. Preventive Veterinary Medicine, Amsterdam, v. 98, p. 39-45, 2011.

86. MARTINS, P. E. Evaluation of potassium diformate on the productive and reproductive performance of broiler breeders. 2005. 88 f. Dissertation (Master's Degree in Animal Production) - Centre for Rural Sciences, Federal University of Santa Maria, Santa Maria.

87. MELLOR, S. Alternatives to antibiotics, Pig Progress, Doetinchen, v. 16, p. 18-21, 2000.

88. MILLET, S.; MAERTENS, L. The European ban on antibiotic growth promoters in animal feed: from challenges to opportunities. The Veterinary Journal, v. 187, n. 2, p. 143-144, 2011.

89. MIRZAIE, S.; HASSANZADEH, M.; ASHRAFI, I. Identification and characterisation of Salmonella isolates from captured house sparrows. Turkish Journal of Veterinary and Animal Science, v. 34, n. 2, p. 181186, 2010.

90. MORAES, D. M.C. Source of infection and antimicrobial resistance profile of Salmonella sp. isolated from broiler farms in Portugal.

cutting. 2010. 66 f. Dissertation (Master's in Animal Science) - Veterinary and Zootechnical School, Federal University of Goiás, Goiânia.

91. MOREIRA, G. N.; REZENDE, C. S. M.; CARVALHO, R. N.; MESQUITA, S. Q. P.; OLIVEIRA, A. N.; ARRUDA, M. L. T. Occurrence of Salmonella sp. in chicken carcasses slaughtered and commercialised in municipalities in the state of Goiás. Revista do Instituto Adolf Lutz, São Paulo, v. 62, n. 2, p. 126-130, 2008.

92. MORITA, T.; KITAZAWA, H.; IIDA, T.; KAMATA, S. Prevention of Salmonella cross-contamination in an oilmeal manufacturing plant. Journal of Applied Microbiology, Oxford, 2005.

93. MOUNTZOURIS, K. C.; PARASKEVAS, V.; TSIRTSIKOS, P.; PALAMIDI, I.; STEINER, T. Assessment of a phytogenic feed additive effect on broiler growth performance, nutrient digestibility and caceal microflora composition. Animal Feed Science and Technology, Amsterdam, v. 168, p. 223-231, 2011.

94. MROZ, Z. Organic acids as potential alternatives to antibiotic growth promoters for pigs. Advances in Pork Production, Edmonton, v. 16, p. 171-182, 2005.

95. MYERS, D. Probiotics. Journal of Exotic Pet Medicine, New York, v. 16, n. 3, p. 195-197, 2007.

96. NAVA, G. M.; ATTENE-RAMOS, M. S.; GASKINS, H. R.; RICHARDS, J. D. Molecular analysis of microbial community structure in the chicken ileum following organic acid supplementation. Veterinary Microbiology, Amsterdam, v. 137, n. 3-4, p. 345-353, 2009.

97. NEGI, P. S. Plant extracts for the control of bacterial growth: efficacy, stability and safety issues for food application. International Journal of Food Microbiology, Amsteram, v. 156, n. 1, p. 7-17, 2012.

98. NIEWOLD, T. A. The nonantibiotic anti-inflammatory effect of antimicrobial growth promoters, the real mode of action? A hypothesis. Poultry Science, Champaign, v. 86, n. 4, p. 605-609, 2007.

99. OETTING, L. L. Plant extracts as growth promoters for newly weaned piglets. 2005. 81 f. Thesis (Doctorate in Animal and Pasture Science) - School of Agriculture, University of São Paulo, Piracicaba.

100. OLIVEIRA, M. C.; CARVALHO, I. D. Performance and carcass lesions of broiler chickens reared on different litter and stocking densities. Ciência e Agrotecnologia, Lavras, v. 26, n. 5, p. 10761081, 2002.

101. OSMAN, K. M.; YOUSEF, A. M. M.; ALY, M. M.; RADWAN, M. I. Salmonella spp. infection in imported 1-day-old chicks, ducklings, and turkeys poults: a public health risk. Foodborne Pathogens and Disease, Larchmont, v. 7, n. 4, p. 383-388, 2010.

102. OVIEDO-RONDÓN, E. O. Technologies to mitigate the environmental impact of broiler production. Revista Brasileira de Zootecnia, Viçosa, v. 37, p. 239-252, 2008.

103. PALERMO-NETO, J. & ALMEIDA, R.T. Antimicrobials as additives in production animals. In: SPINOZA, H.S.; GÓRNIAK, S.L. & BERNARDI, M.M., eds. Pharmacology applied to veterinary medicine. Rio de Janeiro, Guanabara Koogan, 2006. p.641-658.

104. PEDROSO-DE-PAIVA, D. Control of flies and rattlesnakes: Challenges in the poultry production. In: Symposium on Poultry Production Waste, Chapecó, p. 21-27, 2000.

105. PERDONCINI, G.; DA ROCHA, D. T.; MORAES, C. R.; BORSOI, A.; SCHMIDT, V. Presence of Salmonella spp. in day-old chicks marketed for non-industrial production in Santa Catarina. Acta Scientiae Veterinariae, Porto Alegre, v. 39, n. 1, p. 01-03, 2011.

106. PESSÔA, G. B. S.; TAVERNARI, F. C, VIEIRA, R. A.; ALBINO, L. F. New concepts in poultry nutrition. Brazilian Journal of Animal Health and Production, v. 13, n. 3, 2012.

107. PETRI, R. Use of competitive exclusion in poultry farming in Brazil. In: II Symposium on Poultry Health, 2000, Santa Maria. Proceedings... p. 41-44, 2000.

108. PICKLER, L.; HAYASHI, R. M.; LOURENÇO, M. C.; MIGLINO, L. B.; CARONI, L. F.; BEIRÃO, B. C. B.; SILVA, A. F. V.; SANTIN, E. Microbiological, histological and immunological evaluation of broilers challenged with Salmonella Enteritidis and Minnesota and treated with organic acids. Pesquisa Veterinária Brasileira, Rio de Janeiro, v. 32, n. 1, p. 27-36, 2012.

109. PRADHAN, A. K.; LI, Y.; SWEM, B. L.; MAUROMOUSTAKOS, A. Predictive model for the survival, death, and growth of Salmonella Typhimurium in broiler hatchery. Poultry Science, Champaign, v. 84, p. 1959-1966, 2005.

110. QUIGLEY, E. M. Prebiotics and probiotics; modifying and mining the microbiota. Pharmacological Research, London, v. 61, n. 3, p. 213-218, 2010.

111. RAMOS, L. S. N.; LOPES, J. B.; SILVA, S. M. M. S.; SILVA, F. E. S.; RIBEIRO, M. N. Performance and intestinal histomorphometry of broilers from 1 to 21 days of age receiving growth enhancers. Revista Brasileira de Zootecnia, Viçosa, v. 40, n. 8, p. 1738-1744, 2011.

112. REZENDE, C. S. M., MESQUITA, A. J., ANDRADE, M. A., STRINGHINI, J. H., CHAVES, L. S., MINAFRA, C. S., LAGE, M. E. Acetic acid in broiler feed experimentally contaminated with Salmonella Enteritidis and Salmonella Typhimurium. Revista Brasileira de Saúde e Produção Animal, Salvador, v. 9, n. 3, p. 516-528, 2008.

113. RICKE, S. C. Perspectives on the use of organic acids and short chain fatty acids as antimicrobials. Poultry Science, Champaign, v. 82, n. 4, p. 632-639, 2003.

114. RIZZO, P. V., MENTEN, J. F. M., RACANICCI, A. M. C., TRALDI, A. B., SILVA, C. S., PEREIRA, P. W. Z. Plant extracts in broiler diets, Revista Brasileira de Zootecnia, Viçosa, v. 39, n. 4, p. 801-807, 2010;

115. ROBERFROID, M. Functional food concept and its application to prebiotics. Digest Liver Dis, v. 34 Suppl 2, n. p. S105-110, 2002.

116. ROCHA, T. M., ANDRADE, M. A., SOUZA, E. S., STRINGHINI, J. H., CAFÉ, M. B., REZENDE, C. S. M., PÔRTO, R. N. G. Performance and intestinal health of broilers inoculated with nalidixic acid-resistant Salmonella Typhimurium and treated with organic acids. Revista Brasileira de Zootecnia, Viçosa, v. 40, n. 12, p. 2776-2782, 2011.

117. ROCHA, T. P.; MESQUITA, A. J.; ANDRADE, M. A.; LOULY, P. R.; NASCIMENTO, M. N. Salmonella spp. in transport box linings and day-old chick organs. Arquivo Brasileiro de Medicina Veterinária e Zootecnia, Belo Horizonte, v. 55, n. 6, p. 672-676, 2003.

118. ROLL, V. F. B.; DAI PRÁ, M. A.; ROLL, A. P. Research in broiler litter reused for up to 14 consecutive flocks, Poultry Science, Champaign, v. 90, p. 2257-2262, 2011.

119. SAAD, S. M. I., Probiotics and prebiotics: the state of the art. Revista Brasileira de Ciências Farmacêuticas, São Paulo, n. 1, v. 42, 2006.

120. SALAZAR, P. C. R.; ALBUQUERQUE, R.; TAKEARA, P.; TRINDADE NETO, M. A.; ARAÚJO, L. F. Effect of lactic and butyric acids, isolated and associated, on the performance and intestinal morphometry of broilers. Brazilian Journal of Veterinary Research and Animal Science, São Paulo, v. 45, n. 6, p. 463-471, 2008.

121. SANTANA, E. S., ANDRADE, M. A., ROCHA, T. M., STRINGHINI, J. H., CAFÉ, M. B., JAYME, V. S., BARNABÉ, A. C. S., ALCÂNTARA, J. B. Performance of broilers experimentally inoculated with Salmonella Typhimurium and fed diets with addition of lactulosis. Revista Brasileira de Zootecnia, Viçosa, v. 41, n. 8, p. 1884-1889, 2012.

122. SANTINI, C.; BAFFONI, L.; GAGGIA, F.; GRANATA, M.; GASBARRI, R.; DI GIOIA, D.; BIAVATI, B. Characterisation of probiotic strains: an application as feed additives in poultry against Campylobacter jejuni. International Journal of Food Microbiology, Amsterdam, v. 141 Suppl 1, n. p. S98-108, 2010.

123. SANTOS, C. M. R. Effect of using essential oils and microencapsulated organic acids in piglet feed. 2010. 72 f. Dissertation (Master's Degree in Zootechnical Engineering - Animal Production) - Instituto Superior de Agronomia, Universidade Técnica de Lisboa, Lisbon.

124. SANTOS, G. R. J. Probiotics and symbiotics on zootechnical performance and intestinal morphometry of chickens challenged with Salmonella Enteritidis. 2013. 86f. Dissertation (Master's in Animal Science) - Federal Technological University of Paraná, Dois Vizinhos, 2013.

125. SARTORI, J. R., PEREIRA, K. A., GONÇALVES, J. C., CRUZ, V. C., PEZZATO, A. C. Enzyme and symbiotic for chickens raised in conventional and alternative systems. Ciência Rural, Santa Maria, v. 37, n. 1, p. 235-240, 2007.

126. SEGABINAZI, S. D.; FLORES, M. L.; BARCELOS, A. S.; JACOBSEN, G.; ELTZ, R. D. Bacteria of the Enterobacteriaceae family in Alphitobius diaperinus from poultry farms in the states of Rio Grande do Sul and Santa Catarina, Brazil. Acta Scientiae Veterinariae, Porto Alegre, v. 33, p. 51-55, 2005.

127. SESTI, L; ITO, N. M. K. Physiopathology of the reproductive system. In: BERCHIERI JÚNIOR, A.; SILVA, E. N.; DI FÁBIO, J.; SESTI, L.; ZUANAZE, M. A. F. Poultry diseases, 2ª edition, Ed. FACTA, Campinas, 2009.

128. SEIFERT, S.; WATZL, B. Inulin and oligofructose: review of experimental data on immune modulation. The Journal of Nutrition, Amsterdam, v. 137, n. 11 Suppl, p. 2563S-2567S, 2007.

129. SEN, S.; INGALE, S. L.; KIM, Y. W.; KIM, J. S.; KIM, K. H.; LOHAKARE, J. D.; KIM, E. K.; KIM, H. S.; RYU, M. H.; KWON, I. K.; CHAE, B. J. Effect of supplementation of Bacillus subtilis LS 1-2 to broiler diets on growth performance, nutrient retention, caecal microbiology and small intestinal morphology. Research in Veterinary Science, London, v. 93, n. 1, p. 264-268, 2012.

130. SHANAHAN, F. The host-microbe interface within the gut. Best Practice & Research Clinical Gastroenterology, v. 16, n. 6, p. 915-931, 2002.

131. SILVA, L. P.; NORNBERG, J. L. Prebiotics in non-ruminant nutrition. Ciência Rural, Santa Maria, v. 33, n. 2, p. 983-990, 2003.

132. SILVA, E. N.; DUARTE, A. Salmonella Enteritidis in poultry: A retrospective in Brazil. Revista Brasileira de Ciência Avícola, Campinas, v. 4, n. 2, 2002.

133. SILVA, E. N. General control measures for salmonella in chickens. In: COFERÊNCIA APINCO 2005 DE CIÊNCIA E TECNOLOGIA AVÍCOLAS, 2005, Santos, Anais... Santos: FACTA, P. 229-237, 2005.

134. SILVA, C. J.; VARGAS JR, F. M.; SILVA, I. S.; ARIAS, E. R. A.; CARRIJO, A. S.; GARCIA, R. G.; GOMES, R. F. Use of prebiotics (Bio- MOS®) associated with different protein levels in broiler rations, Agrarian, Dourados, v. 1, n. 1, p. 105-116, 2008.

135. SILVA, W. T. M., Probiotics and symbiotics in animal and vegetable feed for broiler chickens. 2010. 54 f. Dissertation (Master's in Animal Nutrition and Feeding) - Marechal Rondon *Campus*, State University of Western Paraná, Marechal Cândido Rondon.

136. SILVA, M. A.; PESSOTTI, B. M. S.; ZANINI, S. F.; COLNAGO, G. L.; NUNES, L. C.; RODRIGUES, M. R. A.; FERRIERA, L. Aroeira-vermelha essential oil as a feed additive for broiler chickens, Ciência Rural, Santa Maria, v. 41, n. 4, p. 676- 681, 2011.

137. SILVÁN, J. M.; MINGO, E.; HIDALGO, M.; PASCUAL-TERESA, S.; CARRASCOSA, A. V.; MARTINEZ-RODRIGUES, A. J. Antibacterial activity of a grape seed extract and its fractions against Campylobacter spp. Food Control, Berkshire, v. 29, p. 25-31, 2012.

138. SPRING, P.; WENK, C.; DAWSON, K. A.; NEWMAN, K. E. The effects of dietary mannaoligosaccharides on cecal parameters and the concentrations of enteric bacteria in the ceca of Salmonella-challenged broiler chicks. Poultry Science, Champaign, v. 79, n. 2, p. 205-211, 2000.

139. TESSARI, E. N. C.; KANASHIRO, A. M. I.; STOPPA, G. F. Z.; LUCIANO, R. L.; DE CASTRO, A. G. M.; CARDOSO, A. L. P. S. Important aspects of Salmonella in the poultry industry and public health. In: *Salmonella - A* dangerous foodborne pathogens. Ed. Barakat S. M. Mahmoud, 2012.

140. TEUBER, M. Veterinary use and antibiotic resistance. Current Opinion in Microbiology, Oxford, v. 4, n. 5, p. 493-499, 2001.

141. TIZARD, I. Salmonellosis in wild birds. Seminars in Avian and Exotic Pet Medicine, v. 13, n. 50, p. 50-66, 2004.

142. THIRABUNYANON, M.; THONGWITTAYA, N. Protection activity of a novel probiotic strain of Bacillus subtilis against Salmonella Enteritidis infection. Research in Veterinary Science, London, v. 93, n. 1, p. 74-81, 2012.

143. TOPPING, D. L. Short-chain acids produced by intestinal bacteria. Asia Pacific Journal of Clinical Nutrition, Neihu, v. 5, p. 15-19, 1996.

144. TORRES, G. J.; PIQUER, F. J.; ALGARRA, L.; DE FRUTOS, C.; SOBRINO, O. J. The prevalence of Salmonella enterica in Spanish feed mils and potential feed-related risk factors for contamination. Preventive Veterinary Medicine, Amsterdam, v. 98, p. 81-87, 2011.

145. USAMI, M., MIYOSHI, M., KANBARA, Y., AYOAMA, M., SAKAKI, H., SHUNO, K., HIRATA, K., TAKAHASHI, M., UENO, K., TABATA, S.,

ASAHARA, T., NOMOTO, K. Effects of perioperative synbiotic treatment on infectious complications, intestinal integrity and faecal flora and organic acids in hepatic surgery with or without cirrhosis. Journal of Parenteral and Enteral Nutrition, Urbana, v. 35, n. 3, p. 317-328, 2011.

146. UTIYAMA, C. E. Use of antimicrobial agents, probiotics, prebiotics and plant extracts as growth promoters in newly weaned piglets. 2004. 94 f. Thesis (Doctorate in Animal and Pasture Science) - Escola Superior de Agronomia "Luiz de Queiroz", Universidade Federal de São Paulo, Piracicaba, 2004.

147. VAN IMMERSEEL, F.; FIEVEZ, V.; DE BUCK, J.; PASMANS, F.; MARTEL, A.; HAESEBROUCK, F.; DUCATELLE, R. Microencapsulated short-chain fatty acids in feed modify colonisation and invasion early after infection with Salmonella enteritidis in young chickens. Poultry Science, Champaign, v. 83, n. 1, p. 69-74, 2004.

148. VAN IMMERSEEL, F.; BOYEN, F.; GANTOIS, I.; TIMBERMONT, L.; BOHEZ, L.; PASMANS, F.; HAESEBROUCK, F.; DUCATELLE, R. Supplementation of coated butyric acid in the feed reduces colonisation and shedding of Salmonella in poultry. Poultry Science, Champaign, v. 84, n. 12, p. 1851-1856, 2005.

149. VESTBY, L. K.; MORETRO, T.; LANGSRUD, S.; HEIR, E.; NESSE, L. L. Biofilm forming abilities of Salmonella are correlated with persistence in fish meal and feed factories. BMC Veterinary Research, v. 5, n. 20, 2009.

150. VIOLA, E. S. Use of acidifiers in broiler diets: residues in the digestive tract and effects on animal performance and intestinal morphology. 2006. 196 f. Thesis (Doctorate in Animal Production) - Faculty of Agronomy, Federal University of Rio Grande do Sul, Porto Alegre.

151. VIOLA, E. S., VIEIRA, S. L., Supplementation of organic and inorganic acidifiers in broiler diets: zootechnical performance and intestinal morphology, Revista Brasileira de Zootecnia, Viçosa, v. 36, n. 4, p. 1097-1104, 2007.

152. VIEIRA, M. F. A. Characterisation and analysis of the sanitary quality of chicken litter made from different materials reused sequentially. 2011. 93 f. Dissertation (Master's in Agricultural Engineering) - Federal University of Viçosa, Viçosa.

153. WORLD HEALTH ORGANISATION - WHO. Risk assessments of Salmonella in eggs and broiler chickens. 2002. Available at: http://www.who.int/foodsafety/publications/micro/salmonella/en/

154. WIEST, J. M.; CARVALHO, H. H. C.; AVANCINI, C. A. M.; GONÇALVEZ, A. R. Inhibition and inactivation in vitro of Salmonella spp. with extracts of plants with medicinal or spicy ethnographic indications, Arquivo Brasileiro de Medicina Veterinária e Zooctecnia, Belo Horizonte, v. 61, n. 1, p. 119-127, 2009.

155. WINDISCH, W.; SCHEDLE, K.; PLITZNER, C.; KROISMAYR, A. Use of

phytogenic products as feed additives for swine and poultry. Journal of Animal Science, Champaign, v. 86, n. 14 Suppl, p. E140-148, 2008.

156. WRAY, C.; DAVIES, R. H.; CORKISH, F. D. Enterobacteriaceae. In: JORDAN, F. T. W.; PATTISON, M. Poultry Diseases, 4th edition. Ed. Saunders, London, 1998.

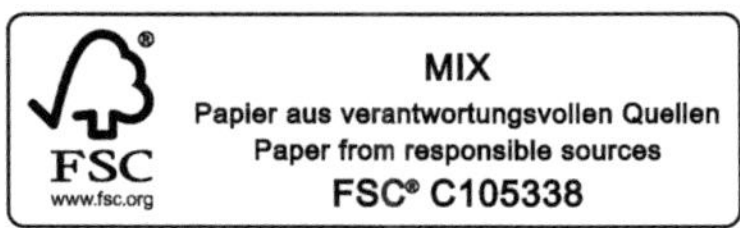

Printed by Books on Demand GmbH, Norderstedt / Germany